# What About the
# Hair Down There?

Published by:
Blooming Twig Books
New York / Tulsa
*www.bloomingtwig.com*

Front cover and author photographs
by Aimee Christenson

Hardcover: ISBN 978-1-61343-072-9
Softcover: ISBN 978-1-61343-073-6
eBook: ISBN 978-1-61343-074-3

First Edition
Printed in the United States of America.

*This book is dedicated to my father,*
*Dr. Arthur Emerson Marquart, D.D.S.,*
*who started me writing young, and despite dementia,*
*continues to teach others through his quiet faith.*

# What About the Hair Down There?

## CHEMO CHUCKLES & TREATMENT TEARS

*One Woman's Story of Family, Friends, Love & Sex*
*After Being Diagnosed with Breast Cancer*

Abby Brown

*"I'm not funny. What I am is brave."*
— Lucille Ball

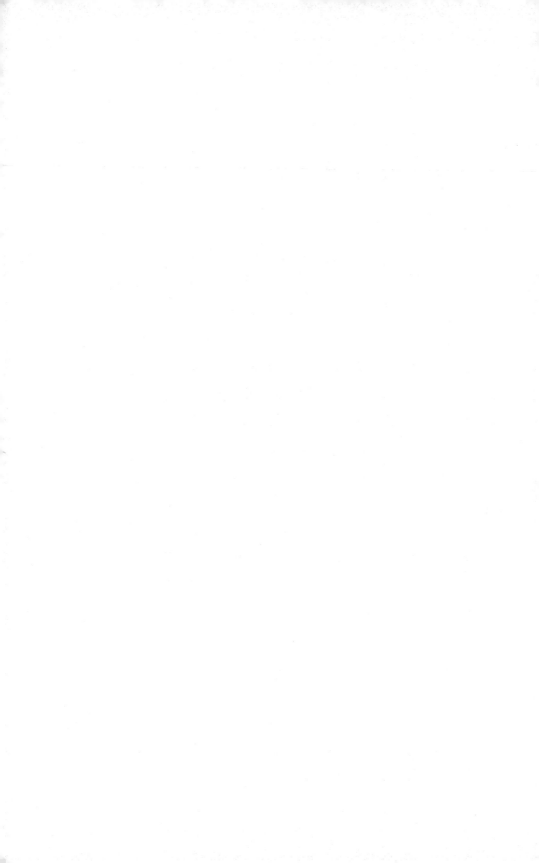

# Table of Contents

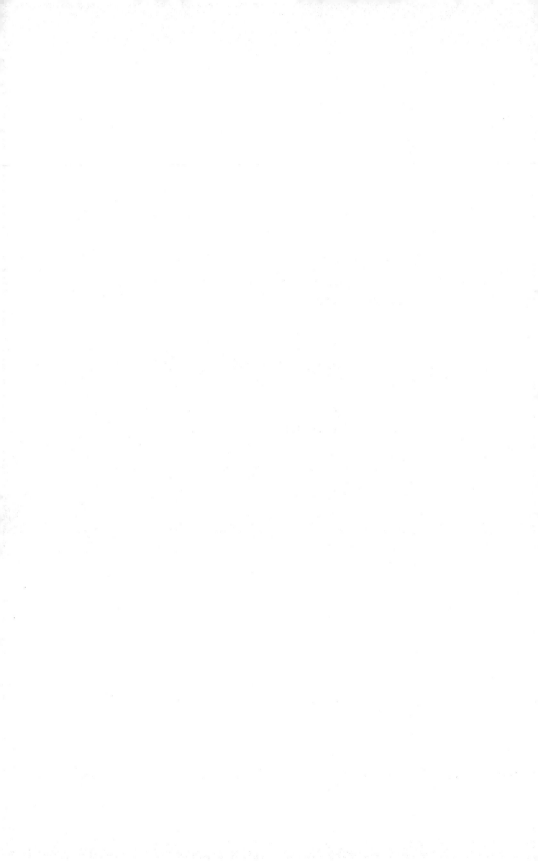

# Introduction

In musing about possible titles for this book, I considered, What About the Hair Down There? At first, it seemed too bold for the front cover, but it was an honest question I had in my own mind as I started the "road trip" of my cancer treatment.

Mine left, like all body hair, and returned with a new look – straight and dark, in contrast to the silver waves that grew back on top of my head. With enough length, some "curl" has returned. I'm not embarrassed to share this with others. It's a fact. And this book isn't *Fifty Shades of Grey*. It's real life.

I'm a mother of two teenage boys, have a wonderful husband of 31 years, and I love my job as a teacher of 25 years at Marine Elementary School in Marine, Minnesota. Add to that mix the family and friends I love I decided to do what I could to stick around a while longer.

This book came about because of encouragement from those who have read my posts on a website called CaringBridge that allows family and friends to participate in the difficult recovery process; writing became one of my solaces during the months of chemo and radiation for breast cancer. I shared thoughts, honest and sincere, regardless of their sensitive nature. And though I knew many people who had been diagnosed with this disease, I really didn't know much about living through the experience of treatment.

As an elementary teacher, I also wanted to educate others on the impact of such a diagnosis on individuals and families. I've been told my words have made people laugh and cry along with me. The journal style is meant to bring about a better understanding of the emotional and physical challenges. It unfolds as it happened – one day at a time.

May this book be a blessing to each of you. It has been quite the "road trip," and it's not over yet. Make each day matter!


— Abby

# What About the Hair Down There?

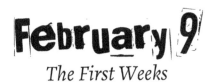

# February 9
## The First Weeks

*"You never know how strong you are
until being strong is your only choice."*

— Bob Marley

On a Friday in early January, my primary doctor found a lump of concern during an annual check-up for my heart meds. With a simple instant message, he requested a diagnostic mammogram as soon as possible. The following Tuesday this was done, leading to a biopsy on Wednesday, and news that confirmed a cancerous breast tumor on Friday. (eight am.)

Because of discomfort in my chest from previous vascular-spasms and various back pains, the following Monday additional tests were ordered: an MRI of both breasts and a bone scan. Both of these were negative for cancer in any other area and allowed me to make the decision to proceed with a lumpectomy. (Simple.)

This surgery took place on January 22. A clear margin around the 1.5 cm tumor was obtained, and the single lymph node they removed tested negative for cancer. We were encouraged and optimistic that treatment of radiation and hormone therapy would be the end of it. (Nope.)

As we anxiously awaited the report from California on tumor specifics, I added in a colonoscopy during my recovery time just in case. My mom's cancerous tumor in her cecum, many years back, put my sisters and me at a higher risk for intestinal cancer. Though I was very aware of the presence of the scope during this procedure (that's another story) these parts were also given a "clean" bill of health. (Wink.)

On February 7, Tony and I made the trip to Regions Hospital in St. Paul for a radiation consultation. At this point, I was debating the necessity of radiation and hoping hormone therapy would prevent future recurrences. Little did we know that this simple option would not even be a consideration later in the day. (Dang.)

That afternoon, the oncologist's appointment provided information that we had not even considered. The HER2 positive, "comedo" ductal tumor was given a high risk rating for 'distant' recurrence elsewhere in the body. This added the word 'chemotherapy' into the necessary treatment plan. We were totally caught off-guard; the box of tissues in the room was emptied as reality set in. The 'nasty' cancer tumor they removed may have sent small cancer cells out into my body, and now they need to be dealt with aggressively. (Crap.)

The journey has taken an uphill climb...I'm getting FIERCE! Thanks so much, to all, for the love and support already given to allow me to proceed with GRACE. Angels watch over us! (Amen.)

# February 10
## What IS vs. What We Thought

Okay – I wasn't going to do an online journal. When my sister, Kris, suggested that I start a Caring Bridge site at the time of my diagnosis, I said, "Nice idea, but I won't need it." Our plans were to get to the simple treatments (radiation and hormone therapy) after the lumpectomy and be done with it. Brain knocking came later!

Things aren't always what we think...perception, hopes, positive thoughts, and faith don't always make what something *is* into what we believe it should be. So, despite all the indicators that the cancer was contained to my breast, reality of the tumor-type straightened out our misconceptions.

Here's the medical scoop:

"Comedo" invasive ductal carcinoma is a higher grade for growth and is more aggressive. Mine is this and was graded a two out of three. HER2 positive tumors grow and spread more aggressively. The tumor removed from my breast also earned this label. (Three out of ten women have this and are treated with Herceptin to block growth proteins from attaching to cancer cells – if they are estrogen positive, which I am.)

Oncotype DX determines a rating score for the 21 cancer "genes" for risk of recurrence. This is done in a California lab. Scores of 31 or higher are considered high risk. My score was a 45, which also indicates a strong "you have no option" outside of chemo. (This number was a turning point for us in our thinking – add, "Shit.")

The combination of all three makes for a 'nasty' case of breast cancer that needs aggressive treatment. One positive is that it is *Stage One* – caught early. Chemotherapy with Adriamycin, Cytoxan, Taxol, Herceptin, radiation, and hormone therapy of Tamoxifen will be used. This appears to be the new 'universal' recipe for success. (I have done my homework!)

My chemo starts on Thursday, February 14. (We learned about my cancer on Tony's birthday weekend and the chemo schedule will land me in the clinic on mine...special occasions are taking on a new twist this year.) It is an every-other-week plan for the first two months, with weekly visits for additional infusions the last eight weeks, totaling four months of intense stuff. Then Herceptin will be infused every three-weeks for one year.

Tomorrow I head back to my elementary school classroom and have to say that I am looking forward to it. I have amazing groups of students to spend my days with, learning together. They will be a wonderful 'diversion.' I am also meeting with members of my new exclusive group: BCB Club (Breast Cancer Bitchin' Club.) I know that the support of women experiencing something similar can make a significant difference in how we live!

# February 11

## A Purpose in This

*"I thought I knew life*
*Touched all the facets*
*Shone in the sparkle*
*Plumbed the depths*
*Clambered back to sparkle*
*I have known life*
*Learnt from experience*
*So why now, this*
*This huge challenge*
*Life threatening?*
*Did I need to look again?*
*Perhaps*
*Could I make a difference?*
*Perhaps..."*

— Carolyn Salter

# February 12

*Prepping*

Today I had a MUGA (Multi-Gated Acquisition) at Lakeview Imaging. It determines the pumping function of my heart's ventricles and established a 'base-line' for mine. This will be monitored over the next year. Sarah and I are becoming friends – this is the third procedure she has done or assisted with over the last month. I told her, next time, I will bring cookies!

I was also treated to a haircut and "adjustment of the grays" by my niece, Cassie, and her colleague, Jessie, who work together at Sassy Di's Salon in Woodbury. These youngsters wouldn't take my money, but I have ways of returning "good deeds." The rate at which hair will exit my head is not known, but I have these sweet girls to help me along.

Spending time in the classroom makes the days go by quickly – I love my job. There is hardly ever a dull day with fifth and sixth graders!

One day at a time – I will be fine. (I am adding that to my signature line on emails!)

Make each day matter.

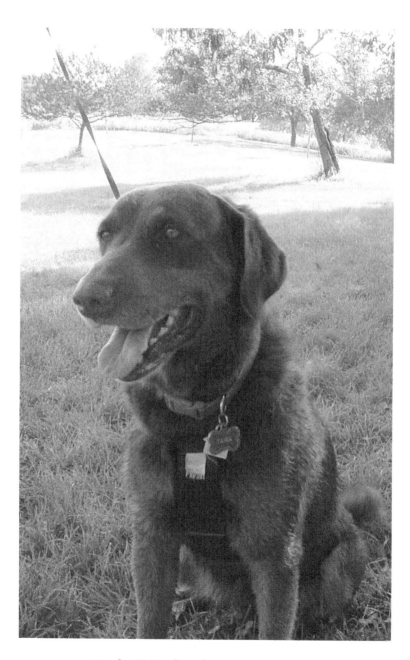

*Our dog Taira, from the MN PAWS Rescue.*

# February 13

*Highs and Lows*

M y son Matthias' confirmation class always ends in small groups that share the week's highs and lows. You know my low...but I wanted all to see our family's *high*.

Taira is a 'rescue' dog...from Tennessee – a chocolate Lab and Doberman mix, about two years old. We adopted her through MN PAWS, and she is a sweetheart! The boys are quickly bonding with her – it is nice to see their "tender sides" come out.

We gave her a pink collar with a pink nametag – she's my girl! She will be a welcome diversion...I am looking forward to the extra company on post-chemo days.

Thanks for all of the well-wishes and prayers. As a team, we've got this! I'll just be viewing things from the sidelines for a bit.

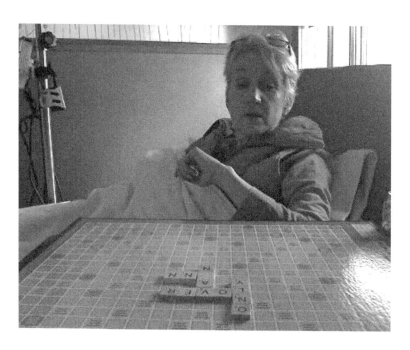

*"Only Lover."*

# February 14
## *Photojournaling*

I've been poked and prodded so many times over the last month that the prep for today's first Valentine's Day chemo session felt like status quo. Most of the time I was able to be positive and share jokes, though it didn't go without the emotional floodgates opening. These will come unexpectedly; we've been told to expect them.

Tony brought a Scrabble Board for us to pass the time. It's an activity we started doing together on one of our anniversary dates and isn't something we find time to do very often between those special occasions.

Ironically, the second word I placed on the board was LOVE. (What is the chance of having all the letters for that?) Tony added an R for LOVER and on my next move I placed down ONLY.

At that time, Tony went to the cafeteria for a bite, and I hit an emotional stage. Despite all of the anti-nausea meds, I was feeling the drugs move through my stomach, conspicuously. It signaled the reality of these drugs as a part of my new challenge. I was not liking the start of the anticipated 'crappy-feeling.'

My nurse, Mary, put on her protective blue coat to administer the chemo. You may not realize that the toilet a chemo patient uses after infusions must be flushed twice with the lid down.

Pets need to be kept out of the bowl – it could kill them. (Yep....add your own thoughts to that one.)

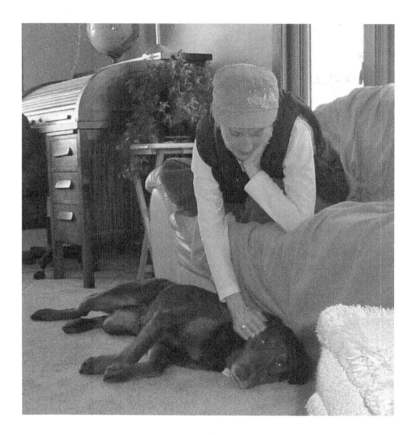

*Bonding.*

# February 16

## *Changing the Karma*

Today, Tony spent time rearranging the bedroom, vacuuming in spots untouched for months, hanging up pictures in new places. I have spent the day hanging low – a bit queasy, but my headache managed by Tylenol ExS. I have my own pharmacy of pills to combat the side effects of chemo and a booster shot for white blood cell generation. (That one causes bone aches.)

Last night, Taira slept out of her kennel for the first time, on the floor next to my bed. It felt protective and symbolic to me. Today, she began making herself comfortable on the couch and was there watching me when I awoke from a nap in the recliner. She spent a good chunk of time outside with the boys today and is settling into the altered life at the Brown's. She's a keeper.

We had company – our dear friends came to visit and make us dinner. Les, too, is a cancer patient – he had a couple years of experience with chemo and stem cell transplants. He made dinner with Tony and only worried us a bit when a steak knife fell onto his toe, cutting it. (Yelp!) He is on blood thinners, so this was not a good thing. Tony doctored him up, and they proceeded to prepare a meal of salmon, couscous, and salad. (Num.) Apparently my taste buds will change as the weeks go by...gotta enjoy one meal at a time and remember to savor it!

We moved an heirloom trunk painted by my mother into the bedroom, and it is now my hat storage and display. Rejoice in creative energy and love that surrounds us! (Hugs.)

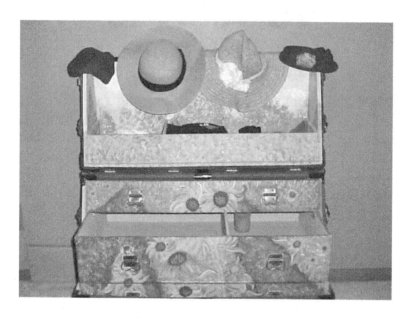

*Trunk painted by Dianne Marquart.*

# February 17
## Temporary "Normal" in PJ's

After a chemo session, somehow eating bon-bons (Valentine's Day chocolates) and reading a novel (or attempting such) while lounging in a recliner (well, dozing) takes on a whole new meaning. I thought about digging out some old movies I bought before Christmas. "Love Story" had crossed my mind, but somehow I wasn't in the mood to watch a woman die of cancer.

And I had this other type of thought today – they say as the hair starts to fall out, go ahead and buzz it off. But what about "down there?"

We enjoyed some spicy chicken chili from a Meal Train delivery today (the recipe has been requested!) I must admit, that is an amazing service and is helpful, particularly when simply moving to the bathroom and dinner table is taxing.

So my taste buds will eventually go, but why is it that my favorite TAB beverage is the first that I notice tasting different? To put it in a mild form of my sister Kris's language: "That kinda sucks."

Tonight, Tony organized the bottles of meds, and put them in their own box. I have some for anti-nausea, constipation, steroids of sorts, a combo drug for anxiety, nausea, and sleep, and need to make a solution to rinse my mouth to prevent sores. I was told to anticipate the Monday after chemo as being the "lousiest." I will let you know.

One day at a time. (Love to all.)

# February 18

## Monday – Mondays

My nurse, Nancy, predicted the Monday after chemo could be the 'toughest.' Though it seems my stomach was better this evening, I do have to admit the morning and early afternoon was taxing and emotional.

Several deliveries of meals were a part of today – one being from my Mom. She and Dad visited for a bit – she wanted to bring along the new hat she knit-up in a day. We are looking for greens to make my eyes 'pop' when I am wearing hats in place of hair. My sister also sent another green one... baseball style. (I am well cared for!)

One hard part of the day was our son Tim's mood. He wouldn't smile for a photo with me...and it made me sad. A picture of me wiping my eyes is on my mom's cell phone. It was real – and I am not going to fake through each day as if *all is okay*. This is hard on everyone.

It is crazy to 'volunteer' to make yourself sicker to get better – but here I am doing it. One does need to be grateful for modern medical advances, along with a jar of Herbal Touch from my friend, Dorothy. (It *will* be ok.)

Tomorrow I see my cardiologist and have minor surgery to have the port placed for easier access to a main vein for infusions and blood draws. One last poke in the arm for that sedative, and my veins can give a sigh of relief.

Your thoughts, prayers, and words of encouragement are soooo appreciated! (xoxo)

# February 20
## De-Lumped Left – The Good Side?

It seems that the procedures for cancer treatment get mixed into the same bag; some are worse than others, but they are "all the same" – crappy. Placing a port into my upper chest area for infusions or blood draws was the way to go – but getting through it wasn't my easiest 'little surgery,' and I wasn't quite prepared for the 'annoyance.' Maybe it was because I couldn't eat or drink from midnight prior and was just coming off my first session of chemo...it made me weaker walking into the hospital than I had been for previous procedures.

You know those little camping cups that "pop open" and close up flat? Hospitals now have a paper sack version to catch the substances leaving your belly after 'upsetting' surgeries. I had the privilege of using one. Being nauseous has gotten old, and dang, it's just the beginning. I may beg for a few of the inflatable tubes for my bedside, just in case they are needed in the days ahead.

Today I stayed home due to the sedative used – no driving allowed – and it was a good thing to be resting and taking pain meds for the new incisions in my chest. It seems the chest muscles were impacted – something I didn't expect. Pushing or pulling with my right arm was not a preferred movement, today.

Taira was disappointed in my inability to do much petting or to take her for a walk. A little TLC for her from the boys did make up for it tonight.

My son, Tim, was the perfect caregiver when he arrived home from school yesterday; he brought me food, beverages, did dishes, and 'tucked' me in at bedtime ... kisses on the cheek included. Matthias, too, was attentive in his own 14-year-old way.

I am still losing some blood via the rectum. Even with the 'clean bill of health' for my colon, it seems that procedure may have irritated the lining. If polyps are removed, bleeding is expected – but I didn't have any. (Watching for this to subside soon.)

As with the others who undergo cancer treatments, I didn't buy a ticket for this ride. There are definitely moments when I want to shout, "STOP! I'm getting off!" It is unsettling to hear the number of women who have 'endured' chemo for breast cancer. Making oneself sick to get better goes against my being! I realize that chemo saves lives, but *chemo does suck.* (And I don't use the "s"-word loosely!)

For now, I am hoping that a good night's sleep tonight, and then time with a classroom full of ten- to twelve-year-olds tomorrow, will perk me up!

# February 21

## *Med Break*

I have a special "chemo-med basket." It is just the cutest container for bottles of "awful" stuff. Thank goodness, it is going to be ignored for the next week!

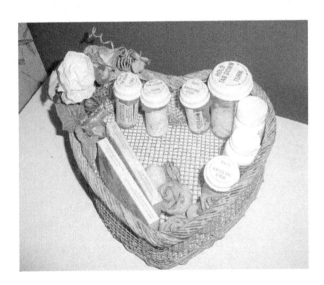

Today brought reprieve. Though I am still dealing with some blood loss and pain from port placement, the hours of the past week have almost been forgotten as I write this post. Amazing, and necessary. In a recent interview, Robin

Roberts, the anchor of ABC's Good Morning America, talked of a total low with her cancer treatment. I get it. And she got through it. (I will, too.)

I work with a group of incredible professionals – real people with hearts of gold. In addition to surrounding me with warmth upon my arrival back to the classroom, they gifted me with future massages – "treatment" that I relish just thinking about! In addition, a parent of a former student walked into the classroom mid-afternoon with a chocolate shake. My students graced me with smiles as they allowed me to indulge in front of them. TLC to the max. (I am blessed.)

And for the next week, I am going to forget that I am a chemo patient. Consider 'no news, good news.'

# February 24
## *When it Rains, it Pours*

**W**ell, for most people the saying goes "when it rains, it pours," but for me, in all my intensity, I am into *monsoon* mode.

I am writing this update from Lakeview Hospital where I arrived at the emergency room last night. I am now minus my appendix. (Fill in the blank with your response to that!)

I started Saturday with what I thought was indigestion. But antacids (lots of them) did not take away the pain. When the diarrhea and vomiting kicked in, I thought it was the stomach flu...only the pain in my gut was different. When visiting my niece at Mercy Hospital, I stretched out on the side bed next to her. We should have taken a picture; she looked better than I did!

Laying down, stretching out, sitting on the pot, doubling over – nothing helped. I finally told my mom I'd leave my van at their place – she needed to get me home, but we stopped for a thermometer on the way to check my temp. It was rising. She headed south and a phone call to Tony had him arriving in Stillwater soon after us.

I love the little community of Marine on St. Croix, Minnesota for many reasons. I feel the same about our local community Lakeview Hospital in Stillwater. As the angels would have it, *my* surgeon for the lumpectomy and port placement was "on call." She watches activity from the hospital on her computer at home and was the one who called the ER doctor to announce I had appendicitis. She was on her way, and though it was later in the evening, she insisted the 'on call team' come in for the surgery immediately. "You don't know what this woman has been through these last weeks!" she told them. God bless Dr. Amy Fox.

I am doing better now and will spare you the details of my morning. She did prescribe taking the week off from teaching to heal – and there will be a 'wait' on my second chemo treatment.

As a friend said to me earlier today, "Someone is swinging you by the tail and isn't letting go!" (Uncle!)

# February 26

## *Fix Me Up*

When I arrived in ER on Saturday, I was in pain and emotionally low. Mom passed me off to Tony (only to return later) and the floodgates opened. But the tears weren't for me; I was sooo sad to be, once again, adding stress/worry into the lives of those I love. As Tony held me, and we cried, his words of reassurance were, "We will all be fine." The *we* is *us*. It isn't something that can be separated out with my *family*.

The morning of my discharge from the hospital, Tom, my anesthesiologist, stopped in my room to visit. He had been 'on call' for my emergency surgery and noticed my low spirits that evening.

Prior to my port placement the previous Tuesday, he shared that his 18-year-old son had been diagnosed with leukemia at the age of one, with recurrence at age three. He had words of encouragement about the upcoming chemo – it is "bad for the good."

He was positive and encouraging, again. His 'volunteer' visit warmed my heart. As he stood before me, I shared that I had thought about his son during my appendectomy stay. It wasn't just meaningful for me to know he is a "survivor," but his story makes real the heartache of parents, friends, and relatives when cancer impacts their loved one. *But* to be responsible for the decision and then *watch* your young child endure 'chemo' – I don't think I could do it...

Tom gave me his card with a hand-written cell number on it. My words of praise for his sincere TLC go along with my praise for Dr. Amy. These professionals model compassion 24/7. (Wow.)

I am including a link to a video from a fund-raising event to support childhood cancer research. Zach Sobiech is a Stillwater-area student. He wrote the song, "Clouds," for his family last fall – it has gone viral. His second release with Sammy Brown, "Fix Me Up," can also be found on YouTube or on Zach's Caring Bridge site. He is an inspiration for finding 'purpose' in our lives = *Now*.

http://www.YouTube.com/watch?v=KvSYZHmhIAM

# February 28

## *A Cut in the Gut*

Some people get "hints" quickly. Some are good at listening to their inner intuition. Others need a swift 'kick in the butt' to hear a message. For me, the 'cut in the gut' was a clear "HELLO!" You can't control and schedule the months ahead....(dah!) Something had to give. This week I had papers filled out for a full-time medical leave from my responsibilities in the classroom. I love my job and am sad to miss time with the students I have grown so fond of, but adding another "Super" to the Superwoman role I share with other women goes beyond my capabilities.

So, I was a 'patient' of interest at the clinic today. An appendectomy? Huh? Seriously?

"Well, I will tell you, it's a first for me," was the comment from my Dr. Corey, my oncologist. As the staff shook their heads in disbelief, they squeezed me into Tuesday's schedule. I will have the weekend to better recoup before my second chemo session.

These past two days, my hair has been 'thinning-out' (including "down there.") A Breast Cancer's Bitchin' Club friend warned me that it would hurt – and it does. Your head feels sore and is sensitive to touch. It must be the follicles opening up and letting go. I will need to make a decision about 'how much shorter' to cut it before having Tony or my niece use the #1 clippers on it.

I have been "banded" many times over the last five weeks. If I were a collector, it would include over a dozen little nametags that have circled my wrist. Since I didn't give Tim, the collector, an option to save them for me, I can't be sure. I don't want these bracelets as reminders of my journey, but I do have a request for those bringing meals. I want to collect *recipes!* There have been so many delicious entrees delivered to our home.

Being surrounded by the love of family and friends makes this endurable.

# March 3

*It's Just Hair – Or is it?*

My hair has often been a topic of discussion when my sisters, mom, and me are together. "You have such a nice head of hair," says Mom.

"Yah, mine's thin and straight," Kris whines.

"Mine, too," Anne chimes in.

Then Kris adds, "No fair."

The hearts of my sister's would not wish my recent 'thinning' on me. And my mom has cried over many parts of this diagnosis, including my pending baldness. I was warned it will be a blatant reminder of the cancer.

Funny, the undetected lump had been a part of me for quite awhile; I felt fine with no outward signs of 'sickness.' Sometimes, ignorance is bliss.

I am also losing my eyelashes – the one thing that gave me the "feminine" look when I've worn my hair short in the past. The little hairs fall into my eyes, poking and making them red. I am debating the need for bothering with a wig – will learn to wrap scarves creatively around my head, but I may have to figure out how to stick "falsies" around my hazel pupils. (So I don't scare anyone when I go out in public.)

When I venture out, now, and see people I haven't met since my diagnosis, I have to respond to the question, "How have you been?" I forget that the news can be upsetting for them. If they can hold it together, I can, too. But if tears sprout from their eyes, I am a puddle. Today was the first time I have been to church in over a month. It was exhausting. I knew enough to skip the mascara and load my pockets with Kleenex.

I have a husband who is afraid to kiss me for fear I will get sick. We are going to have to have a serious talk with my oncologist to reassure Tony that I am not a porcelain doll. Not being able to share some skin with the man of my life for these next four months will make this even more unbearable!

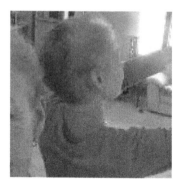

*Thin or sparse – what's the difference?*

# March 4

## *A Better Day*

Today I visited my students to reassure them that I will be in for special projects and on my 'good days' to assist with the annual Marine Elementary 6th Grade Play. I spent the night with my parents, so while I read student journals this morning, Mom made chocolate chips cookies for them (Sugar Mama Marquart at it, again.)

My students were a bit 'stunned' last week to learn I would not be returning, but today we all made it through our circle time without tears. The best part was when I went to leave. One of the students announced, "Time for hugs!" Each one gathered around to give me a sweet embrace. This is an example of why I didn't decide to take a full-time medical leave from the start. I love these kids and my job at our small community school.

There was quite the hair loss today when I took a shower and then combed my head. People say they lose it after the second chemo, but it really only takes one infusion of that poison to cause this. I did my best to do a 'bald guy' cover-up before heading to school; long wisps over the sparse spots. The girls looked through the American Cancer Society catalog pointing out the hats and wigs they liked the best. I purchased a few more hats at Herberger's, and alerted my niece, Cassie, that the buzz cut would be needed tomorrow.

I have taken a few pictures of my thinning hair and shared them with the Caring Bridge community. The hair loss is temporary, which is more than most "guys of age" can say. I know it is just hair, but have been warned it is always a bit of a shock to lose it via chemo. I can't pretend baldness will come without tears, but I will do my best to smile.

Tomorrow is my second chemo session. Despite extra emotions yesterday, I have had some days of 'feeling good.' My stomach is healing well – I even took the dog for a short walk. I didn't realize how many times my appendix was 'acting' up until its removal. No 'false' indigestion or gut discomfort since! Come mid-summer, I will be a new woman.

(One day at a time – I will be fine!)

# March 6
## Minus Hair – Still Smiling

The much-anticipated buzz cut took place after a 'breakfast for dinner' fixed by my sweet niece, Cassie. We sat down as a family with her and her fiance, Tom, to eat before she took out her clippers. By last evening, the hair that remained was scattered about my head in wisps. While Tom ran the camera on his iPhone, Cassie proceeded with care. My head was sensitive and sore, but she was gentle.

We have always known I am my father's daughter, but the proof is in the bald spots. I have a similar birthmark above my left eye that Cassie said he has on his! On our next visit together, I will get a pic of our heads side by side.

A March snowstorm closed area schools yesterday, but Tony and I were determined to get to the clinic for my second chemo treatment...we are keeping this show on the road! The room was packed, and it made me comment that it is downright scary there are so many people (men and women) who are undergoing this medical treatment. Lakeview is just a small facility – and this was just one day of the week. Bad weather didn't keep us from receiving infusions. (Crazy.)

There is a topical numbing agent to use prior to the procedures that I am going to try – just to take the edge off the needle poking into my skin. I was also blessed with a volunteer who gifted me with a Healing Touch session. Gayle is a retired Stillwater School District nurse – an exuberant soul with positive energy!

I am also grateful for the follow-up days of anti-nausea drugs and don't want to imagine what this was like prior to their availability. I need a injection to boost the production of white blood cells today. The boys are joining me for a ride into town.

My son, Matthias, didn't hang out in the kitchen during my buzzing session. At the time, he took a quick peek of my bare head, then said, "Okay, you can put your hat back on." Earlier today, he took the picture of Tim and me, but would aim and turn his head to snap. He announced that he wouldn't be going to Gamestop with me, unless I have something to cover my new do.

My son Tim on the other hand, told me this morning, "It doesn't look that bad." He is concerned about my head being cold when I don't have it covered. I do have to say that when a five-minute-heat-wave comes upon me now, I am unzipping my sweatshirt and whipping off the hat! For those who have experienced the effects of menopause, you will understand when I say, "Hot flash, my ass." Heat wave of five minutes is a better description.

# March 9
## *The Buzz on Video*

People who know me, know I am not a 'couch potato.' But, I have dubbed myself a 'lounge veggie' during these post chemo days. That's a positive twist to lying around most of the day, wouldn't you say? The recliner serves me well for 'vegging' out – it's a necessity to rest after the poison has been infused into my system. (Bluk.)

I am tracking side effects, and am in the "hang low days," but have been blessed by visitors who bring meals, provide pleasant conversation, and clean (Thanks, Mom – I know the hair was a bit much in my bathroom!) Matthias and Tim have been on spring break, so there has been a bit more action around the house. Taira hasn't gotten as many naps as usually, either, but digs the extra attention. I have plans to get her out for some good walks next week. This dog doesn't know that I do more than make frequent trips to the bathroom and level myself out into my chair.

We published Tom's video of my Buzz. It took a bit of reading and learning to figure out how to get it onto YouTube; thankfully I am not into full 'chemo-brain' on top of accelerated menopause. It's about twelve minutes long, and is an invitation to experience a bit of this small breast cancer event with me.

https://www.YouTube.com/watch?v=97cwvEHjxUM

I will post a second one of Cassie's 'styling' me up with scarves tomorrow. I have received more hats – some for sleeping, some for show, and some to 'cover-up' as directed by Matthias.

Enjoy the smell of melting snow! I am waiting for the sound of our first bluebird.

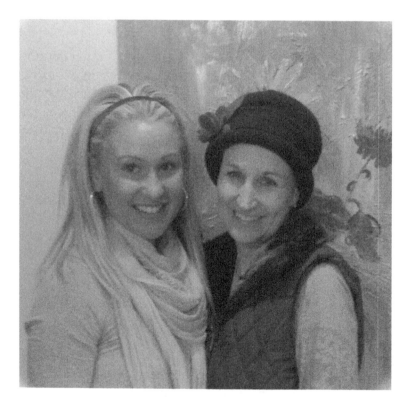

*Cassie, the stylist, AKA sweet niece.*

# March 10
*Sharing Gifts Video*

Early in our days together, I learned that Tony and had I different preferences for shower temperatures. When more than cleaning-up was involved, it was easy enough for me to adjust to 'cooler' as things 'got steamier.'

But, my own body, alone in the water, is confused these days! I start in with the test on my arm, then continue to immerse my lower half, but as soon as I tip my head back – too hot, then BRRRR! I never realized what a buffer hair was in water! I've already got the hat thing going, but this showering scene has me grabbing the towel fast when I am finished. I need to get the moisture off of my top half quickly, so that I don't have an extra-cooling effect taking effect over the rest of my hairless body!

Yesterday, taking a shower and doing a bit of light housework and picking-up had me in tears – it was frustrating to feel so wiped-out by it. Hopefully by chemo treatment #3, I will better understand this, so that I am not putting unrealistic expectations on myself. Today, I showed signs for turning the corner toward the better 'between' days. Church, taking a drive to visit my folks, and grocery shopping was enough, though. I was told that being fatigued is not the same as being tired. I get it, now.

The cards and well wishes that continue to come my way are daily reminders of the kind hearts we all have to share – for the good of our world. There is so much we can't control in the craziness and behavior of others, but just for today, we can work to make our own neighborhoods a better place. Smile, say kind words, and be thankful for the gifts God has given us! Make each day matter.

Here is a video of Cassie fixing me up:

http://www.YouTube.com/watch?v=mPQym6QvSxA

# March 12

## *Super-Surgeon Dr. Amy*

It could be said, "It's all in a surgeon's hands." But in my case, *my* surgeon operates with *heart*! Dr. Amy Fox and I have recently been sharing 'our story' regarding the number of times she and I have frequented the sterile room together. Yesterday, during my post-op check-up for the appendectomy, she counted the number of incisions she has made on my front half in the last month = seven. As we went over the report that stated the appendix was simply infected, I mentioned I still have my gall bladder. "No more surgeries!" was her response.

This young woman is not only a gifted surgeon, but has the bedside manner of an *angel*. How can you not love someone who works to heal you with gentle hands, laughter, tears, and hugs?

I am moving into my 'good week.' Food tastes good, fresh air is invigorating, and my energy is returning. I still have to remind myself that I can't do as I am used to...as the chemo works to kill any possible cancer, the rest of me works to stay alive! (CRAZY!)

So, this is proving to be one of the most difficult challenges I have faced in my lifetime – and there have been a few. I can't say the day went without tears; chemo also makes you emotional, but having time to reflect is important. I can keep my mind occupied with talk shows, cooking shows, and books, but do know quiet is needed to gather strength to face what each day brings. I don't know how anyone could go through something like this without some kind of faith. I believe there is a greater purpose, whether we understand it at the time or not.

May you delight in the small wonders of our universe, knowing there are no words for what is beyond our earthly world. (Hugs!)

# March 14

## Bad Hat Days

It may sound funny but, now instead of bad hair days, I have bad hat days. I am still trying to figure out what is comfortable to wear out in public. Some itch, don't match my outfit, aren't warm enough, or just plain look dumb. I have been gifted with many soft ones, knit with love by my aunties and others, but I am using those for hanging around the house. One of my sister-in-laws posted she thought the scarves are 'sassy.' (I am trying to get all over that look!) I may not have to dry any hair, but am finding it takes a little extra time to get out the door with the right touch on top of my head!

When I am 'out and about,' I am adjusting to glances from people. They don't stare; but there is the recognition that I am wearing a hat or scarf as a cover-up of something BIG (and BAD.) Sometimes you can sense they are rooting for you through their extra-warm smiles. I bet I could even get to the front of a long line via someone's goodwill gesture – like those extended to little old ladies. I want to feel normal, but am realizing I have to adjust to a 'new normal' for a while. Eventually, I'm sure, it won't feel strange. And hopefully, when someone asks, "How are you doing?", I really can be okay.

This week, the salesclerk at Herberger's inquired as much, sharing that she was a registered nurse. I was exchanging a pink HOPE bracelet, and my hat was sliding sideways, too big for my now-bald head. I thought I was okay, until she asked. (Dang.) As I tried to formulate an answer, I realized I wasn't, and tears brimmed my eyes. Hers filled, too, as I simply told her I have had two cycles of chemo so far. Her encouraging words are what most say, "They can do so much for cancer these days. It will turn out fine."

It was a good day. Taira and I had a 30-minute walk down our country road, and for the first time in a long time, I got a bit sweaty from something other than a five-minute heat wave. The air was fresh, and the morning snowfall covered up the mud from yesterday's thawing. The bluebirds are smart enough to stay south for the time being, but the spring chirping of the chickadees promises an end to this long winter.

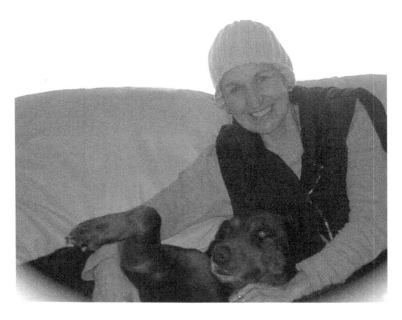

*Something to smile about.*

# March 16
## Comfort – Food, Dog, Family, Friends

There are days when a bowl of mashed potatoes with butter or gravy just hits the spot. One day, I made a box of macaroni and cheese, almost polishing off the entire pot by myself! When my sisters and I were little, recovering from the stomach flu, Mom would fix us toast and hot green tea with milk and sugar. Lately, I am enjoying cocoa chai with honey and milk and am becoming a hot-chocolate snob. It's the simple things that can bring a smile and a sigh. I am in the 'good days' between chemo. And feeling "well" never felt so good!

Taira has become the ultimate cuddle-dog. She goes from one person to the next to be scratched and played with on the floor or outside, finally exhausting herself into a nap. She has bonded uniquely with each of us. During the week, she is my watchdog – even pushes open the bathroom door to find me when I leave the room. (so much for privacy!) If I sit on the couch, she takes it as an invitation to snuggle on in. She is another kind of comfort. In sickness and in health, dogs don't need to take a vow!

I continue to be overwhelmed by the warm wishes, prayers, and acts of kindness that come my way from family and friends. It isn't surprising, because my life is filled with amazing people, but it is humbling.

Yesterday, a friend posted the following in my Guestbook online.

### Five Tips to Giving Life All You've Got
*Carol Moehrle*

1. Be kind. Every day.
2. Smile. Put on a happy face and keep moving forward.
3. Find your passion and strengths. Find meaning in the work you do.
4. Forget regret. Leave mistakes and regrets in the past and move on.
5. Be grateful. Say "thank you" to all those who affect your life positively.

(View this day as a gift and give it all you've got.)

# March 18
## *The Talk (R-Rated)*

I love my Breast Cancer's Bitchin' support group. We try to meet weekly; and that's what is needed when you are in the throes of treatment. What "The Gals" have told me is they feel good 'giving-back.' You see, I am a 'newbie' and when I've cried out – they've been there – all 'survivors' willing to share their breast cancer experiences. Bless their souls!

Today's topic of (my) concern was...S.E.X.

Remember when I mentioned I was going to ask my oncologist about 'skin time.' I did. Her response was, "Sure – go for it – whatever feels good. But, just so you know, as with the possible mouth sores, you can also be a bit sore down-yonder." (OK – thanks for the warning?)

What the majority of you may not know is that chemotherapy puts you into accelerated menopause (in addition to the other side-effects, most of which I don't want to read on the drug reports.) And as a result, those 'parts' get as dry and cold as a desert at night, and yep, sore. The youngest member of the BCB group reported her solution, "Don't do it!" The older members gave advice that included getting 'some stuff' from the pharmacy.

I have to say, in 30 years, we've never needed 'any stuff' to help us out. (Pretty darn good, wouldn't you say?) And let me tell you, I never knew there were so many options of 'that stuff' on the shelves! Jeepers – I don't know if I made the right choice, but want to have something on hand – just in case the urge overtakes the reality that it's now a 'sensitive' endeavor that needs to be pursued with caution.

(Damn.)

# March 21
## *Close Lid – Flush Twice*

I am back to the practice of closing lid and flushing twice – I also close "my" bathroom door for a week after chemo. (Three down – five to go.) I have to share, many days after my first infusion, Tim forgot and used this bathroom. He came into the kitchen in a panic, rubbing the back of his thighs. "Mom, I just sat on your toilet! Should I take a shower?" As he danced about, I reassured him that it had been enough days of flushing and simply sitting on the seat wasn't going to harm him. Poor kid – the worries abound around here! (Hey, the thought just occurred to me that this stuff could be a sort of Draino for the pipes out to the septic tanks. What do you think?)

I've added other pictures to my online photo album. There is one that shows the 'red stuff' going in. (FYI- it comes out pink.) And an update on Scrabble – Abby 2, Tony 1. My first word: QUEEN. (smile.)

A couple of stories come to my mind as I head into the clinic every two weeks. One is of a colleague who sat on the bed as her contractions started for the birth of her second child. She looked up at her husband with tears in her eyes and said, "I don't want to do this, again." (Yep, but ya gotta.)

The other is from my childhood. Mom was dressed-up to go somewhere, but first, my sisters and I needed some kind of vaccinations. When we arrived to the clinic on that Saturday morning, the place was quiet. I remember just the nurse with the needle, and my sisters and I running around the waiting room screaming and crying, "Nooo!" Lord knows how she ever stuck each one of us, but let me tell you, the fumes were coming out the window of the car as Mom drove us home. We were lucky to be alive as we slipped into our bedrooms and closed the doors – grounded.

Mom can be proud of me, now. I'm behaving like a big girl. Tony drops me off at the front door, before parking the car, and I walk myself into the clinic. No kicking and screaming – just doing what is needed to stay alive.

# March 23

*Heat Waves*

I don't realize I am doing anything, but as my son Tim hangs with me, he asks, "Having a heat-wave?" I had just frantically and quickly unsnapped my down vest – a standard to keep me warm. He's always been attuned to people and their behavior. I had to laugh, because I was. I asked him how he knew, as I grabbed for my knit hat. His reply, with a sheepish grin, "Because you rip your clothes off!" Well, not all of them. It starts with my prayer shawl being tossed off my lap, knee-high wool socks pushed down to my ankles, and then I lay back to feel the furnace burst from my internal parts to the surface.

When some childhood friends and I spent time together in Las Vegas last November, we saw "Menopause, the Musical." "Burn, baby, burn – disco inferno," takes on a whole new meaning at this stage of the life-game. The *heat* is another side effect accentuated from the chemo and especially bad at night. Guys on chemo get them, too. Imagine that!

So my friend, Toni-from-the-Marine-Garage, mentioned she could smell the chemo when we hugged and cried the other day. Now that it's been mentioned, I think I notice it, especially if the scent of my lotion has worn off. If I really want to find out how 'bad' it is, I can ask Tim. He's also the honest one about stuff like that. This will be another topic of discussion for my Breast Cancer's Bitchin' support group.

Matthias sat down on our bed to chat a bit, too, while I hung out in my "other recliner" in our bedroom after school. It was to first remind me that I owe him his allowance from Sunday, and then we found some things to laugh about.

"How was school?"

"Good. (smile)"

Nice. He didn't realize I was without a hat (result of an earlier heat wave.) That is a first – he has always told me to "cover-up" in the past. Progress of some kind – acceptance, I'd like to say. Later though, when he stopped in to say goodnight and give me a hug, he said he'd let me kiss him – with the condition that my then-covered head didn't touch him. (He's 14... Still, I love these boys of mine!)

I visited school, too, and got hugs from all my 6th graders. Remember, I had asked the girls to choose some hats and wigs from the American Cancer Society's TLC catalog for me to consider...I got my list from them. I am actually doing well with scarf-variety and am skipping the wig. I still need work on 'the stylin' to get out the door, though have a few more months to get it perfected. But then, I have learned to let go of some of the perfectionism of my youth...and that is not a bad thing. Who knows, by the end of this chemo scene, I may be heading out the door with my birthday head!

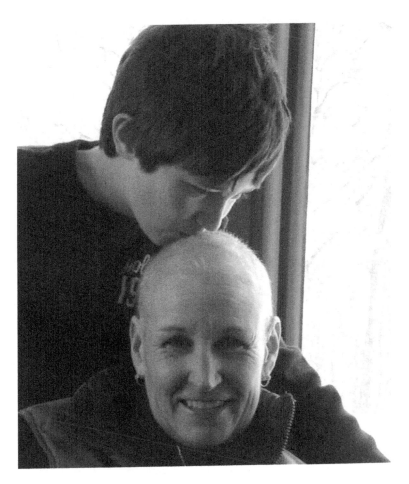

*Unconditional love.*

# March 26
## Chemo-tose vs. the Three-Day

My head continues to be confused by what it needs to be comfortable and warm. I grew up in Superior, Wisconsin. In all those years, I don't recall *snow* this late in March. So when I have ventured out for short jaunts this week, I still need the winter hat, but feel a bit foolish wearing one in public. I've learned to have a 'car hat,' and then do a quick switch, before exiting out the door. I have also realized that fashion scarves are not correct for wrapping well around the head – there are 'head scarves' for such. Geez, between 'winter weather in March' and a 'chemo head,' this is all a bit complicated! The orbit of our planet around the sun is inevitable, though...this will all pass. (Thank God.)

I have come up with a term to describe the days immediately following infusions: *chemotose*. (A blend of chemo and comatose.) It is a state that allows for minimal functioning. Expecting no more than taking a shower, getting a few dishes washed, running one load of laundry, and pushing the remote to switch TV stations is realistic. Taking naps and lying in bed with my laptop helps pass the time. I try to keep the anti-nausea drugs to just three days. They can cause constipation (despite pills to prevent it,) and I spend proceeding days dealing with that 'accumulation.' The 'booster' shot for stimulating white blood cells causes bone aches. My muscles have never had so much rest...Lord knows how they will react when I can be serious about a 'fitness plan' again! The dog is patient with waiting for these days to be done in each cycle; we will be trekking together soon... We've got bluebirds to spot!

A post on Facebook announced that my niece, Cassie, and sister, Anne, have committed to walking the Susan B. Komen Three-Day Walk this summer in my honor. I continue to be brought to tears by the gestures people make in support of this challenge. Their goal is $2,300 each! I now have a goal to walk alongside them for whatever my 'post treatment' body will allow, come August!

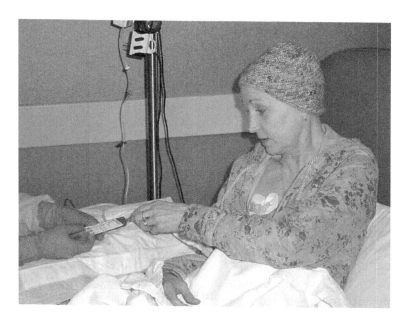

*Beware, the Red Devil.*

# March 29

## 54 and Still Kickin' (Temporarily Lower)

My 54th birthday, on March 28, was a delightful one. It started with a visit to school. There is something undeniably heartwarming when you hear kids call out your name with enthusiasm, "Mrs. Brown! We're so glad you are here!"

We did a birthday activity break *and* an ice cream treat. We also started an art project, then I attended music class with them for the announcement of parts in the upcoming sixth grade play (School House Rock.) When I dropped off ice cream for my 5th graders, I received the same sweet response. (I love these kids!)

I also enjoyed lunch at a local establishment with a dear friend. As small as the towns of Marine and Scandia are, we have our pick of good places to eat. After that, I needed to renew my driver's license. I am sure you know what worried me – my headdress! I kept it simple – black 'breast cancer' scarf. It will be a five-year reminder of this fight to be cancer free.

People use the saying "I felt like I was going to die" loosely. When the term comes to my mind to describe a situation, I now consider its seriousness. In the afternoon, my heart was a-pumping hard, and I was extremely winded. Why? I joined a group to dance the "Cha Cha Slide," many times, for a Power-Up promo video. Many of you know this song with directions to "slide to the left, (move) slide to the right (move) stomp right one time (stomp) and so on... It's not that hard, really. Well, unless you have had chemotherapy, which can impact lung and heart functioning, and you haven't done more than walk the dog for a 'cardio-workout' the past two months. (Geez!) It's foreign to me to feel so breathless. I was glad a couple of phy -ed teachers were also 'dancing.' I knew their CPR skills were up to date! For me, being active is a part of my 'real' lifestyle. This is a temporary one I'm living. I may be kicking low, but I am still kicking!

The day finished with carry-out (dinner) and cake. I was in bed early – and too brain/body exhausted to think about writing this post. I am into my 'good days' of this cycle and looking forward to MANY HUGS at our open house – birthday and life celebration tomorrow!

Our hearts beat for a purpose. Find yours!

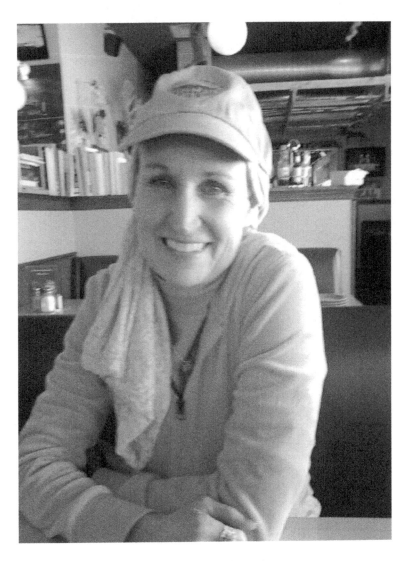

*Sporting the new hair-do.*

# April 1
## Special Needs Patient

Of my many years in the classroom, the most recent ones have professionally stretched teachers to use data to meet the learning needs of individual talents. We have a wide spectrum of children and do our best in the 'group' setting to make this happen. In the world of education, this is called differentiated instruction.

I'm not sure what you call it in the medical field. But I continue to challenge my surgeon, Dr. Amy, with unique situations to handle. I have dubbed myself her "special needs patient." I write this journal entry from Lakeview Hospital where I am spending some time, again. The diagnosis is mastitis – a big, bad infection of the boob! It hurts horribly and is being treated with warm compresses, plus two kinds of antibiotics via IV, over the next couple of days. My temp is up, as is my white blood cell count, which means my body has been working to fight the infection. I couldn't do it on my own, though. Discharge to be determined.

A couple of the gals from my BBC support group came down with pneumonia, but mastitis for breast cancer patients is *rare*. Yep. Here I go again! I am going to have Tony pick up a couple of lottery tickets for me = the *odds are in my favor*. (Tongue in cheek.)

Dr. Amy and others continue to shake their heads. Chemo has been postponed. Being on medical leave not only makes sense when people are going through treatment, but has become a necessity for me. Working to beat the cancer and deal with whatever else comes my way is a full-time job!

Despite my aching breast, we did have a delightful Easter weekend. The cake and ice cream social I planned, followed by our extended family March birthday dinner, was a natural high for me. The wide variety of visitors included past and current school families, neighbors, relatives, and friends from childhood to those from Marine. But my college friend, Dori, gets the award for driving the furthest, three hours one-way from La Crosse, Wisconsin. It was a surprise trip and had us both in tears! So much for the fresh make-up I had put on! We have not seen each other for 20 years...but friendships of the heart are timeless. It felt like we had just been together. What a wonderful day! I was in bed by 8:00 p.m. – exhausted and happy. :-)

The capacity to love is amazing – there is no limit. I continue to be filled with incredible warmth, from my tippy-toes up to my bald head, by the care and love of the people in my life. I am so blessed!

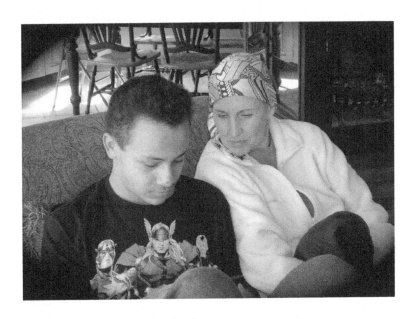

*Simple moments.*

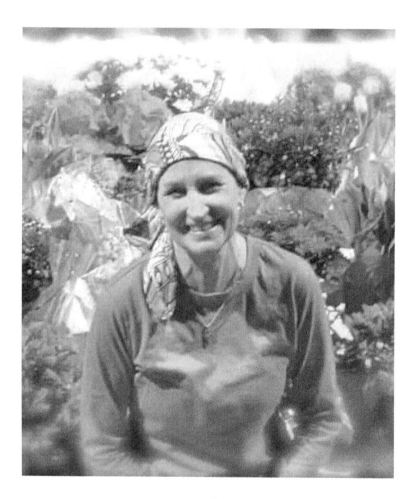

*Easter Sunday, 2013.*

# April 3
*I'm Still Here – Lakeview Hospital*

Just to educate a few, I have learned that mastitis typically occurs with breast-feeding due to cracked or irritated skin. Nipple piercing can also lead to mastitis (who in their right mind?!) In my case, the incision from the lumpectomy wasn't fully closed yet, and so was an avenue for 'normal skin bacteria' to get in and grow. (Crud.)

When my sisters and I were "developing", we complained about the genes we seemed to have inherited with regards to "women parts." Mom would reply, "Be glad they're not bigger. They just get in the way, and you can't button your shirts."

I can tell you that this week, I am glad I only have a little more than a good-sized handful to swell up! Several friends responded they have had mastitis during breast-feeding and, along with an oral antibiotic, were told to continue using 'that side' with the baby. Hold onto your seat as you imagine the infant latching onto the nipple of a swollen breast filled with milk *and* infected mammary glands! (Oh, good Lord!)

I am spending a third night at the hospital. Because I am not lactating, the inflammation and infection is slow to move-out, even with two types of IV antibiotics round the clock. My compromised immune system is also slowing the process of healing. This needs to be dealt with before I can have my next chemo. It is frustrating; I am almost to the halfway point of my treatment. Tomorrow I will most likely have another ultrasound to see if there is a 'pooling' of fluid that could be aspirated out with a needle. Worst-case scenario, Dr. Amy will need to take me back into the operating room to lance the sucker. (Okay, now who is saying "ouch?")

For tonight, the nursing staff is going to help me get more than 3 hours of sleep in one stretch. The many interruptions for vital checks and IV's have me heading into that of a nursing mother who functions on naps – sleep deprivation is not helpful for healing, either!

"I will be fine – one day at a time." (Repeating that one many times this week.)

# April 4
## Knight in Shining Armor

*"I know God won't give me anything I can't handle.
I just wish he didn't trust me so much."*
— Mother Teresa

**M**y Knight will be arriving after supper to rescue me. Good thing I am on the first floor as I don't have any hair to hang out the window! Prayers and better rest along with the bags of antibiotics seemed to do the trick last night – finally. By morning my flaming red breast had calmed down and my white blood cell count had dropped to almost that of a 'normal' person. My incision is almost healed shut. Dr. Amy was elated and went skipping out of my room at 5:30 a.m.; I would have joined her, if I hadn't been hooked up to the IV bag! I have an appointment with the oncologist tomorrow and most likely will have infusion #4 on Monday.

Chemo patients have a special pass into ER or clinic with a temp of 100.5 Fahrenheit. I am not the only qualifying cancer patient being cared for in a hospital room at Lakeview this week. I have said it before, and I have reason to say it again – I love our small town health care facility! They could use the "Cheers" theme song for some of us:

"Dah, dah, dah, dah, where everybody knows your name." The food has been good – healthy – lots of spring mix greens and fresh fruit to add to the entrees. I even have been able to get bottles of ice tea and lemonade to make my own Arnie Palmers. Because the beds can be remotely adjusted for support under the knees and also incline, I have to admit they are more comfortable than some in hotel rooms. I did bring my own pillow, but can say my 'stay' has been pleasant. Really.

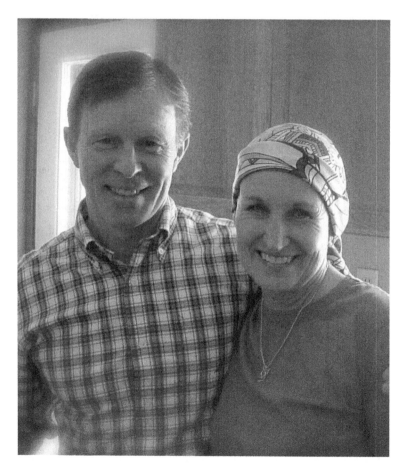

*My knight.*

# April 7

## *Healing with Faith and More*

At the cake and ice cream social I had pink COURAGE bracelets for people to take home. There were some left in the bowl when I drove myself to the hospital on Monday, but I noticed they were not there upon my return home on Thursday. Later on, my son Tim said to me, "Mom, you know those bracelets? I hope you don't mind, but I brought them to school for some of my friends. They said to tell you to get better soon, and they are thinking about you." Geez – of course it was OK, and it completely touched my heart. Twelve-year-olds can be amazing.

As I recover from the mastitis with much less pain and redness, I've been informed that the 'hardness' will take some time to soften. I now have a 'perky' breast with an unmatched partner that hangs low. Not that anyone else will notice when I put on the proper "going out in public" attire, but it does make for an interesting look in my lounge-wear!

When I am done with radiation, the repair work needed most likely will be to reduce and lift the untreated side to match the 'damage' done to the current perky one. Crazy. My first day in the hospital, it did cross my mind that I had a choice to do a single or double mastectomy...and I had a fleeting thought that I should have just 'lopped' the bugger off! You know, this whole breast cancer thing has all kinds of pain involved, regardless the treatment. Deep breaths, faith, love, and support from all gets me through this *path* I am on.

The incision is slowly closing – and my oncologist, Dr. Corey, said she could reduce the strength of the chemo this next round. Two major infections that my body couldn't fight off are enough. I am now two weeks off from the original plan, but learned early on that this breast cancer treatment stuff doesn't follow a schedule. Tuesday is the appointment for treatment #4.

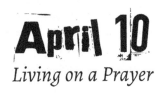

# April 10

*Living on a Prayer*

*"Oh-oh, we're halfway there,*
*Whoa-oh, living on a prayer."*
— Bon Jovi

For those of you familiar with Bon Jovi's hit "Living on a Prayer," you will now have it stuck in your head as a reminder to say an extra one for me!

Yesterday's chemo session took longer to get labs results back from the blood draw, which made us a bit nervous coming from my hospital stay. I did some quick talking to my angels, and thank God, all turned out to be in the 'acceptable' range to go ahead, so we are officially done with four of eight bi-weekly infusions. The final two months will change to drugs called Taxol and Herceptin. I will be going in for the heceptin weekly, but apparently it is a short session. In years past, women would have been done at this point, but research has shown improved reduction of recurrence rates with the additional two drugs, thus the longer treatment. I will still have radiation, making this entire 'battle' a six-month process. It's what you do in my shoes, though.

I am reading Deanna Farve's book, *Don't bet against me! Beating the odds of breast cancer and life*. She and Brett were not married in college when they had their first daughter. Deanna was a single mom for the first years; she lived the life of a struggling young woman trying to make ends meet and at one point quit college to work full time and pay the bills. This life experience lead her to HOPE Foundation that provides financial support to single mothers who have been diagnosed with breast cancer. Many don't have insurance plans that cover all the costs or any insurance at all.

The day after each chemo infusion, I've mentioned there is an injection given to boost your white blood cells. In 2005, when Deanna saw a bill for medical expenses covered by their insurance, the cost of this Neulasta injection was $3,000 for one shot!

I have had many surgeries, hospital stays, chemo and the upcoming radiation...I can't imagine how people with no medical insurance would even be able to consider getting the treatment they need. I am fortunate to have good medical coverage, but it breaks my heart to think of the struggles other endure to 'stay alive.' Thank goodness for those like Deanna, who are able to create foundations to assist. Her strong faith has helped her with public appearances to share her story; she is shy, but believes all things happen for a reason (as I do).

Our local paper ran an article online. The title has me as a "former teacher." I want to reassure everyone, I will be back in the classroom come fall!

(Cancer be gone!)

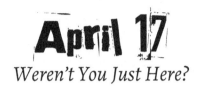

# April 17

*Weren't You Just Here?*

Yesterday I checked in at Lakeview Hospital for imaging of my heart. The receptionist's comment, "Weren't you just here?"

Well, actually it's been two weeks since I checked in for my hospital stay, but maybe seeing anyone more than once a month qualifies as becoming a familiar face. At least she still needed to ask my name to register...but with the many procedures I have had since early January, my average is two per month.

Next week I will start the new chemo drugs, so a new baseline was needed to be sure no damage was or will be done to the ventricles. The amount of blood pushed out from my left ventricle is the same, and although I feel as if I can hardly breathe with some activity, it is functioning well. Part of my fatigue comes from low hemoglobin. No matter how well I eat, the chemo keeps it down. Along with the "One Day at a Time" mantra, I find myself daily repeating, "It's only temporary. It's only temporary."

Which is more than I feel I can say about *winter* in Minnesota this year. It is April 17. The temp is in the mid-30's. Healthy people are having trouble dealing with this...it is not good for the emotional health of anyone! I don't want to wear winter gear to walk the dog anymore. It is taking some extra effort to stay out of the looming depression, but I am working on it! Getting out of my pajamas and the house for even part of a day can help.

And it doesn't matter how old you are, sometimes you still benefit from a little "mothering." I am fortunate that my parents live close; I can pack a bag for a spontaneous overnight with them. Changing the scenery has helped to keep my spirits uplifted on my 'good days' with this gloomy, cold weather. I take my time running errands and even plan a 'sit-down' lunch if I venture out...all by myself. It's a different kind of quiet time. I remember when the boys were little that even being able to go to the grocery store without them was a treat! As social as I am, even chatting with complete strangers at times (just like my dad – and to the embarrassment of my children,) I have to admit there is a new silence I need to keep in my head. Additional outside 'stuff' coming at me interferes with that.

Overstimulation can cause meltdowns in little ones – no different for people on chemo! Being "edgy" is also something I am more often ... I try to warn the family, especially at night, so they can prepare for any potential "bite" coming their way. The smart thing for them, stay away from Momma when she moves into that mode!

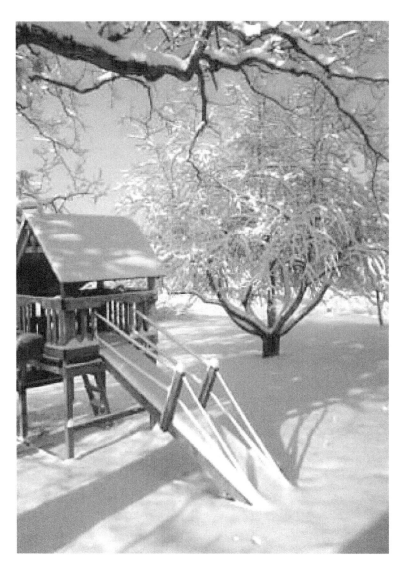

*Endless winter.*

# April 23

*Phase Two – New Chemo Drugs*

In February, when we started the chemo scene, thoughts of the two-month mark put green grass, spring flowers, and warm breezes into my mind. On this late April day, we had inches of new snow adhering to the trees and on the ground. Once before, Tony maneuvered his car through snow-covered roads to the clinic for a treatment. However, today the roads were not a problem. We arrived on time at 9:00 this morning. The challenge this time was different; it was patience.

There were four new chemo patients and the pharmacy had an unusually great number of 'individual cocktails' to mix and deliver. Even without delays, this new bi-weekly infusion regimen will be a six-hour visit. The Taxol drip takes three hours. Herceptin is 30 minutes. There are two prep bags of liquids that contain four different preventative drugs for side effects and another one with saline solution; it all adds to the time I sit in the blue chair. And it also requires many more walks with "my bagged friends" on the five-wheeled-stand to the bathroom – all strings attached. (Flush twice – close lid.) . Scrabble update: Abby: 4, Tony: 1.

My son Tim commented again today that after chemo, my eyes look red and "scary." He pointed this out last time and is correct. All that stuff going in seems to seep out wherever possible. My eyes water more after infusions. That is not listed as a side effect for the drugs. The steroids given to increase appetite rev you up – thus the night owl hours when I write after a day at the clinic.

I will do the follow-up shot tomorrow to boost the white blood cells and need to return next Tuesday for a 30-minute Herceptin infusion, thus I will be in clinic weekly for either the 'works' or this 'quickie.' Herceptin is the drug that women continue for one year after completion of initial treatments, if they are HER2 positive. Then there is the pill I 'qualify' for, and remember, radiation for a month or more is a part of the package. Honestly, it could be called overkill, but kill it we must. (I am not interested in doing this again!)

I have to admit, I have had a bit more anxiety about the potential side effects for this new batch. It has received mixed reviews from my Breast Cancer's Bitchin' support team. In 6th grade, I teach a unit on Newton's Laws of Motion. One experiment has students push down a little rubber headed animal onto a rubber suction cup – compressing a spring between. They then place them on a desk – and wait. Most of you know what is suppose to happen; eventually the critters will fly into the air. But not all of them do, and it can't be well predicted. It's an individual thing. And even the same unit could react differently on the next trial. Put my head on a spring and push it down onto a suction cup – that's how I feel tonight. I can't say what is going to be my reaction to the stuff my body was infused with today. But, I'll keep you informed on what pops up!

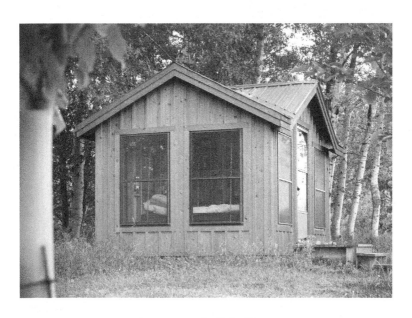

*A sanctuary built by Tony.*

# 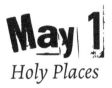May 1

## *Holy Places*

A couple of years ago, the theme of Pastor Joel's sermon was "personal holy places." One of mine is the bunkhouse Tony built that sits on a high spot of our acreage. It is made, in part, with wood that he planed with his dad in Wisconsin and that dried in our pole barn here in Minnesota. It is the last place the sun shines as it sets and is surrounded by poplar trees that whisper in the wind. Tony also built two swinging beds and a storage box for bedding. On one of our warm days this past week, I cleaned the windows and floor and was finally able to spend my first night of the spring season being lulled to sleep by the sounds of the leaves and frogs peeping. Excuse my reference to the demons below, but it has been a hell of a long winter. I am grateful for this little sanctuary out back; it allows me to feel connected to the higher beings of our universe at what seems to be a 'mid-treatment' crisis.

Yesterday was an emotional day. I hadn't expected it. I have had a cough and drainage from my sinuses since my hospital stay and earlier this week noticed a sore throat with ear pain kicking in. When I was little, I had many ear-aches. Mom would warm a small bottle of medicine in a pan on the stove, and I recall anticipating the liquid as she dropped it into my ear with a love/hate of the feeling of the drops moving down into the canal. The heat felt good; the crackling sound was icky. The ear hurt horribly, and I'm sure I would cry. I haven't had an earache since my tonsils were removed in 2nd grade, until this week.

I was scheduled for a Herceptin infusion and had plans to have lunch with a close colleague, so added an appointment to see Dr. Williams mid-afternoon, the doctor who had found my lump on January 3. When Tony and I met with my oncologist, Dr. Corey, she said, "Not to be melodramatic, but he may have saved your life."

I hadn't had a chance to tell him thanks and found myself weepy on the way to Stillwater. It's been just shy of five months since my diagnosis, and there are several more months of treatment to go. Half-over is not done, and things were feeling like a long haul. By the time the nurse set the needle into my port, I was flowing a river. (Geez.)

As the angels would have it, the retired school nurse from my district was doing her volunteer rounds for "Healing Touch." And again my teaching partner of 23 years decided to drive to the clinic for my infusion before we went to lunch. The three of us worked out my tears recognizing that they were needed. I will say it again, it has been a hell of a long year. (Can I cry, "Mulligan?")

By the time I sat in the examining room to see Dr. Williams, we were able to reflect on the episodes of the past months without any tears on my part. When I shared the oncologist's comment and said, "Thank you," he was humble and took his next diagnosis seriously. I do indeed have an ear infection and the start of bronchitis, both caught early. It seems that if he had seen even the slightest tinge of pink in my ear, he would have put me on an antibiotic, though. You don't take chances with a chemo patient who has a compromised immune system. He gave me the reminder to go directly to ER if my temp reaches 100.5 degrees, then added his notes to my lengthy log in his computer.

This latest mix of chemo drugs does not cause nausea for me, which is a relief. I have had some acid reflux, the heat waves are intensified, and I do experience muscle and bone aches for the first several days, mostly in my hips, guts, lower back, thighs, shoulders...well, I guess any are subject to an ache. I attempt to do push-ups and hold a plank, but muscle strength has also taken a hit. I also can forget that fatigue is still a part of this and have forged forward with daily tasks until I am exhausted, too quickly, by too little. Naps still needed. My eyebrows and eyelashes continue to thin, as well as "down there," though I just learned that this particular 'look' is 'in vogue' with the younger generation. Somehow it doesn't have the same sex appeal for a 54-year-old with breast cancer and a bald head.

I am signing up for a free workshop called, "Look Good, Feel Better." It will be a chance to spend time with more women enduring chemo treatments. And I still rely on my BCB group for support. One recently gifted me with her "chemo doll." I was touched. The prayers and endless kind gestures from so many keep me taking it one day at a time.

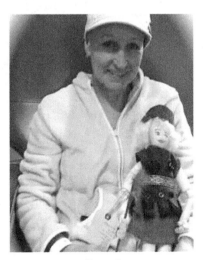

*Tenacity.*

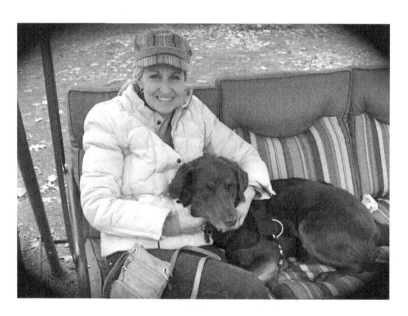

*Loving life at the lake.*

# May 7
## Six Down, Two Biggies to Go!

Tuesdays are 'chemo' days for the next five weeks; some infusions take longer, but only two will be Taxol/Herceptin days. A Scrabble update for you; Tony came back with a win today, putting him at 2 to my 4; it was needed for his ego. (He's gotta bring in two more wins for a tie breaker.)

The biggest annoyance today has been a gut ache – not nausea, but what leads to acid reflux. I am trying to get on top of it with stronger antacids. I am expecting muscles and bone aches over the next several days. Dr. Corey did say I should be able to be more successful with longer dog walks and other activities to get back into 'shape.' I'll still need to monitor how much to 'push' in a day to avoid fatigue and exhaustion.

The warmer weather is a lift for everyone's spirits in Minnesota. Today I planted flower seeds inside the perimeter of our fence of the new raspberry garden. Everything will harvest later this fall; we still don't have apple blossoms. But, there is more light from the sky, and I see a light at the end of the chemo tunnel!

When I arrived home from the clinic, there was a gift bag with our mail near the door. It didn't have a card, so I was concerned I wouldn't be able to thank the 'giver.' The mystery was solved when I lifted out a t-shirt with a postal stamp imprinted on it...one that supports Breast Cancer research. Our neighbor is the post-mistress in Scandia where mail is sorted for delivery in our area. My name and Toni-from-the-Marine-Garage were included on the back. It was a heart-touching gift.

My mom knitted me a pair of socks with the breast cancer ribbon... (the cutest things ever?!) My aunties continue to knit 'cool' hats for me. I will have to do some modeling of a few, along with spring scarves and hats I've been finding at thrift shops and on sale elsewhere. I've decided I want to 'start anew' with my wardrobe and am putting many of my old clothes into bags to share with others. Anything I've worn for more than a few years, or not at all in a few years, are on the way out the door!

I attended a modern dance performance in Minneapolis with some my fellow teachers last week. We had dinner first and arrived home late. (FUN!) Another one of the 'gifts' this medical leave has allowed is more time with family and friends, especially those I haven't seen in a while. When Mom needed to go 'up north' last week, I took my dad out for lunch, to a half price bookstore, and then we both napped and spent time sorting through a box of old photos and news clippings. His dementia has him forgetting current things, but he loves to talk about the days gone by. I am grateful for days like this with special people in my life.

This weekend we will 'open' our unit at Mallard Lake Family Resort near Webster, Wisconsin, and reconnect with our summer friends. This is another 'holy place' for me. The park model we have is comfortable and provides rest for the soul. My radiation schedule may alter the amount of time spent there this summer, but I hope to get a couple mid-day stays in during the month of May.

I have a young man named Zach Sobiech in my thoughts today. His bone cancer is becoming difficult for him. This past week he attended prom with his girlfriend and celebrated his 18th birthday. His story is one of incredible faith. Watch the following video, and be sure to have tissues on hand.

http://www.YouTube.com/watch?v=9NjKgV65fpo&sns

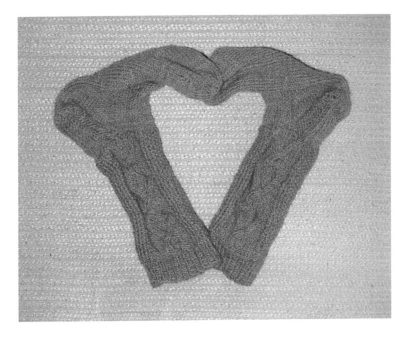

*Breast cancer socks by Mom.*

# May 21
## Number Seven of Eight and
## Trying to Look Good to Feel Better

I am really beginning to see a dim light at the end of this tunnel. Today, I marveled that even when one is enduring something like chemo, weeks pass at an amazing speed, if you live it 'one day at a time.' While teachers and kids count down the days remaining for this school year, I am looking ahead to the final chemo celebration in two weeks. Though I still have radiation for a chunk of the summer, I may be going 'hat and scarf-less' to school this fall!

This new combo of chemo includes the addition of Benedryl to my pre-meds. It prevents any possible allergic reaction to the drugs – though I get a flushed reaction for part of the next day. It also guarantees a nap during the six-hour procedure. But first, the Scrabble game takes place. Last week Tony added another win to his tally giving him a chance to tie the tourney today. I have to say, our words have become a bit more sophisticated with a few even being two syllables. We use a Super Scrabble board with "quadruple letter" opportunities on the outer edges. Though Tony was ahead the majority of the game today, one of my very last plays was QUIT on a "triple word" line – a 39 pointer pulling me ahead of his 26-point lead. The nurses always get a chuckle out of our competitiveness and quietly cheer me on. So, this tournament is mine – 5 to 3. I foresee a challenge to a new round of 8 games beginning in two weeks!

I took along my handcrafted Warrior Doll to the treatment today. Her name is Tenacity. "Not easily dispelled or discouraged: persisting in existence or in a course of action" is the computer-dictionary's definition of this powerful word. Seems like a fitting description for this new doll of mine, and describes many of the people with whom I hang! (Thanks, again, Chemo Sister Julie!)

Since my last post, I attended the workshop offered by the American Cancer Society. A handful of women being treated at Lakeview spent a couple hours together. A cosmetologist led us through a 'make-up' lesson using a bag full of free goodies. We used humor with one another – despite our chemo challenges. I learned how to add lines to my disappearing eyebrows, and apply eyeliner to my top lid (this was quite humorous!) My eyelashes used to outline my eyes for me. With eye shadow applied all the way up to my partially fake eyebrows, I can pull off 'looking good' in public. I am telling you, though, as the remaining hairs on my face disappear, my son Matthias may not only tell me to 'cover-up' my head around the house. He may request a full-face mask.

I was the only woman to bare her bare head at the session, which I found a bit sad. One shared that she even couldn't look at herself in the mirror without hers covered up. Even though people reassure those undergoing chemo that inner beauty matters most, most women would admit that glamorous gowns and diamonds can't even make you feel better in public, if you are having a bad hair day. Really, think about it. All the same, I am working on the guts to say, "The hell with it; I don't care what people think." Members at Mallard Lake Resort may have to get used to my new look this summer, and so will Matthias.

These next five days will be managed with non-narcotic drugs for the aches and pains and will include a 'flushed' face tomorrow, along with a cleaning out of the digestive system. Though I don't feel nauseated and fatigued, I need to remember that my heart and muscles are not strong enough to deal with the chemo and much additional 'activity' this next week. Last week I was able to get Taira out on a couple 'long walks' which used to be my old 'short walk,' so I know I can plan on that next week. I was a bit frustrated when my legs could only hold up for one fast dance during a girls' weekend last Saturday. My childhood friends all understood my need to sit out the "next one," though. Again, I had to remind myself it is just temporary.

We all have our life's challenges. We are mourning the loss of Zach Sobiech who exemplified that living a long life is not necessary to do good on earth when you have a Heart of God. His story was recently featured in People magazine:

www.people.com/people/article/0,,20701996,00.html

Make each day matter. (Love to all.)

# May 27
## *Prayers for the Tooth!*

I need to be honest and share that not every day goes by with a totally positive attitude on my part. The day after my last chemo, I had a melt-down. The word QUIT on the Scrabble board rang from my mouth as I announced to those in the clinic reception area I would sign the papers that released them from being responsible for my health – I was taking it into my own hands. Like a ranting two year-old, the tears flowed, and I declared I wouldn't be a guinea pig in the world of breast cancer treatment.

Let me back you up an hour or so. On my way to the clinic for the follow-up shot (the one to help white blood cell production,) I called Regions Radiology Department. We needed to know how to 'restart' the process for scheduling radiation and wanted info for the New Richmond, Wisconsin option. During my conversation, the gal on the other end commented that I would need to schedule a new consult with the radiologist there; he may not have the same 'treatment plan' as the doctor at Regions. What the heck? Yes, she said, he would be able to see what was recommended in my records from January, but he might want to do something different...

Now rationally, I realize, this may mean only a 'tweak' in the plan, but she was talking to a woman filled with chemo – the seventh of eight, mind you, and I wasn't in the mood to hear 'variations' were even possible. There was also a comment that he may not agree with her thoughts on whether I can have the Herceptin chemo during the radiation treatment... Stress level rising....

Then, at some point during the drive to Stillwater, I grabbed the last piece of red licorice between the seats from a bag that had been there awhile. After tugging off the first bite, I chomped onto something harder than the licorice. My tongue discovered the hole that the 'tooth' piece left behind. (Super damn.)

In January, on the same day the Dr. Williams found the lump, I had visited the dentist to do a temporary repair job on a tooth that needs a crown. It hasn't been done; chemo doesn't allow major dental work. And it is the same tooth, but another part.

As I write, I don't recall if losing the new piece of tooth occurred before or after my phone call, but by the time I walked into the clinic, I was at the peak of frustration. When it was confirmed that the radiation would most likely be a 'standard' five times per week for six weeks – 30 zaps – I couldn't keep it together. "I'm done. I've had it. I'm tired!" (Whaaaaaaa!)

Of course the nursing staff watched my flowing tears and listened with caring ears and hearts. And a fellow-chemo patient looked at me with pleading eyes and said, "You can't give up, now."

I'm not. But it is taking some time to adjust to the reality that the majority of my summer ahead will be consumed with daily trips to the clinic...40 minutes (one way) from Marine, and 90 minutes (one way) from the lake.

As far as the tooth goes, our local dentist did a temporary "magic construction" with some goop, and I am using

Tim's ortho wax to cover a little sharp edge. I am making an appointment for three weeks from now – a two-week wait after my last chemo. In the meantime, we need to pray the thing doesn't abscess, which would mean I would need a root canal!

I also completely 'let go' of any involvement with the Marine 6th grade musical this year. It is in wonderful hands with other professionals, but I had hoped to work with the kids a bit. Again, I expected too much of myself, and added this sadness to the tears this week.

Okay – enough whining. The "poor me" bellyaching won't help with healing. This is an emotional battle, too, but I will 'get over it and get it done.' I have much to be thankful for with a good medical policy and days available that don't involve working part-time with a part-time substitute teacher for the classroom.

Tony, the boys, and I enjoyed a wonderful Memorial Day weekend at Mallard Lake. The kids and dog are exhausted from hours on end of activity. I have taken a couple naps, and Tony is into a good book. He and I even shared the same bed two nights in a row (to guarantee a good night's sleep at home, we have a 'separate bedrooms' arrangement.) It's been months since my 'need for stuff' post – and I will simply share it was tried out for the first time this weekend. (Yep, poor guy. Life with a wife on chemo calls for many sacrifices.)

We have been reconnecting with the delightful families that make up the resort and who are our cherished 'summer friends.' The boys and I may be detouring through Somerset to get here some weeks, but we will make it happen. It is a place that allows us to step back in time a bit – Tony references it to the life on Mayberry RFD...simple and sweet.

Indigo buntings, Rufous-sided Towhees, and Rose-breasted Grosbeaks have arrived back to our yard. I am expecting serious summer weather, soon!

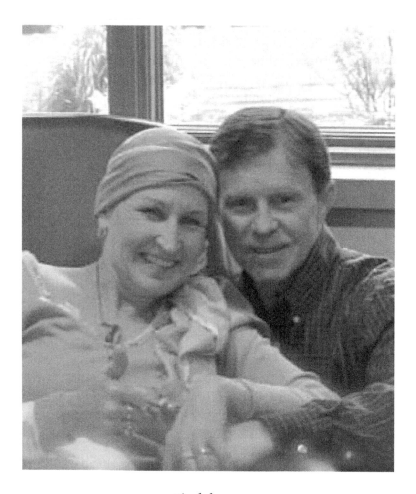

*Final chemo.*

# June 5

## *Done with the Big Ones!*

Today's chemo treatment #8 was done in five hours – record time! These last four infusions of Taxol and Herceptin are given via separate drip bags. Tony and I skipped the Scrabble game. The Benadryl given in pre-drips (along with three other bags with a steroid, anti-nausea, and saline solution) put me out for most of the three hour Taxol treatment. But I am extra-fatigued for many reasons. I attended all performances of the 6th grade musical last weekend and a hospital stay for my Dad may have compounded the other side-effects of months of chemo.

Awhile back I posted about *chemotose* – a word I actually made up to describe the vegetative state caused by the fatigue/nausea of Cytoxan and Adriamycin. Now I appear to be moving into the cumulative effect that leads to what they call *chemobrain*. It can be temporary, though sometimes lasts up to a year or more, and once was blamed on other things like hormone changes and aging. It's now recognized as a result of chemo treatment alone. (Shit!)

What is chemo brain? (from the American Cancer Society)

- Forgetting things that they usually have no trouble recalling (memory lapses)

- Trouble concentrating (they can't focus on what they're doing, have a short attention span, may "space out")

- Trouble remembering details like names, dates, and sometimes larger events

- Trouble multi-tasking, like answering the phone while cooking, without losing track of one task (they are less able to do more than one thing at a time)

- Taking longer to finish things (disorganized, slower thinking and processing)

- Trouble remembering common words (unable to find the right words to finish a sentence)

Today's dose has moved me quickly into dealing with muscle aches and stomach acid. And get this – the bottom of my feet hurt horrible – as if I have been standing on them for days. I haven't. How ironic is that for someone who wants to get back at walking ASAP?! Here is a reminder to you and me; just another week for most of these side effects. As long as I don't forget how to get home while driving or hiking in the months ahead, all is well! ;-)

Tomorrow I will be playing the usual teacher-role for a 6th Grade Recognition Celebration. Their performances of School House Rock, Jr. Live! were fabulous last week, improving noticeably from the first to the fourth performance. It is difficult to fathom how the months have gone by so quickly since I 'left them.' When I was diagnosed with breast cancer in January, the end of the school year seemed an eon away. Even when dealing with illness they have seemed to melt away.

The students gifted me with one thousand paper cranes during the dress rehearsal last week. It left me in tears and speechless on stage (for real!). The love that went into each fold filled my heart. I am sooo blessed!

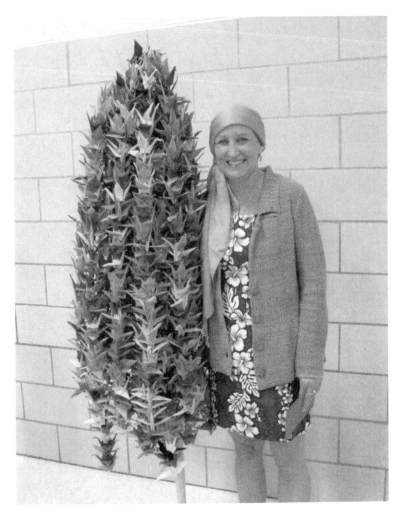

*Origami cranes — Marine Elementary.*

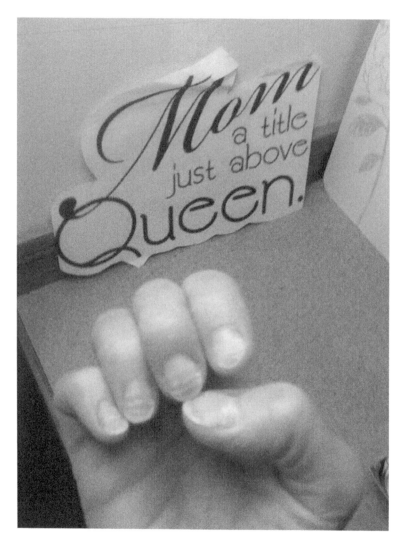

*More side effects.*

# June 12
## Uncharted Mosquito Territory

Breast cancer patients have many things in common. There is an instant bonding that occurs when you meet another having had or currently in treatment. I can share something that I don't think many chemo patients have experienced, though. First of all, I live in a state where mosquitoes thrive on summer nights. And when I sleep out in the bunkhouse, I have to use the toilet nature provides – one surrounded with trees and green grass. So, dear friends, picture this: A woman is baring her bottom to empty contents of the bladder in a squat position, something her weakened leg muscles don't appreciate. You need to know that this individual is accustom to swatting near her back-side to keep the skeeters from taking a bite, but quickly realizes that due to chemo and hair loss, there is new exposed skin available. The 'down yonder' spot is free and clear to the varmints of the north woods. Her arms are a-swingin' and her legs are aching as the job is finished. When she collapses on the swinging bed, she spends the next 20 minutes dealing with a brain sending signals from her aching feet to her itching privates. Good Lord, and angels above, somehow she falls asleep with prayers for fast healing of all parts! (Yep, adventures of Abby – as good as they get these days!)

Though the drugs are meant to kill the cancer cells, other body parts also take a hit. My fingernails are short, soft, and streaked with white spots. You have to consider the trade-offs in the deal. New nails will grow, along with my hair in the months ahead...happening one day at a time.

Since my last post about my last "big" chemo, bigger side effects kicked in than those of my previous Taxol infusions. Yes, my feet hurt soon after, but the pain continued into a new intensity that I had not experienced previously. I thought I was in the clear, and was feeling unjustly smug about it, but Taxol has a cumulative effect that I hadn't anticipated (and now have been made acutely aware!) I have only said this once in my previous entries, though it is a common phrase, "Chemo sucks." There, I have made it doubly official in my book.

Neuropathy is a common side effect of many things besides chemo including diabetes, alcohol abuse, shingles, low vitamin B levels, and some autoimmune disorders. The following information is from the American Cancer Society web site specific to the impact of Taxol and other chemo drugs on neuropathy. I now understand why I have been dropping things and have been experiencing a handful of the other symptoms listed, in addition to the specifics on nerves.

What are the symptoms of CIPN?

The symptoms or signs of chemo-induced peripheral neuropathy (CIPN) depend mostly on which nerves are involved. The most common symptoms are:

- Pain (may be there all the time or come and go, like shooting or stabbing pain)

- Burning

- Tingling ("pins and needles" feeling) or electric/shock-like pain

- Loss of feeling (can be numbness or just less ability to sense pressure, touch, heat, or cold)

- Trouble using your fingers to pick up or hold things; dropping things

- Balance problems

- Trouble with tripping or stumbling while walking

- Pressure may hurt more than usual

- Temperature may hurt more than usual (mostly cold; this is called cold sensitivity)

- Shrinking muscles

- Muscle weakness

- Trouble swallowing

- Constipation

- Trouble passing urine

- Blood pressure changes

- Decreased or no reflexes

In summary, CIPN can cause severe pain and can affect your ability to do things like walk, write, button your shirt, or pick up coins. If it gets very bad, it can cause more serious problems like changes in your heart rate and blood pressure, dangerous falls, trouble breathing, paralysis, or organ failure. (Geez.)

The most 'stressful' for me was definitely the foot pain. It didn't matter if I was lying down or standing – the bottoms of my feet ached increasingly for about five days. The worst of it has seemed to pass, and Dr. Corey, Lakeview Oncologist, said it should continue to get better, but tingling can last weeks into months. One from my Breast Cancer's Bitchin' Club said her feet are still numb. I guess I can be grateful for the feeling of pain!

I am foregoing narcotics, as I have in the past, and switched to a generic form of Aleve to use with the extra strength acetaminophen. Apparently there is a pain med that targets nerves, but I will skip that, too. Walking the dog any distance is out of the picture for a while longer, but I do have to remain optimistic about improvements.

Tony and I met with the radiologist in New Richmond, Wisconsin, last week. Radiation will begin the last week of June for 6 ½ weeks – 33 treatments in all. I can't say I didn't let the tears of frustration flow as we talked, but the combined chemo and direct zaps to the breast are a layering affect that has proved to reduce recurrence to around 5% from 30% with just chemo (in my specific case). Big girls do cry, and then get over it. We were told to expect the same "tiredness" I have been experiencing with chemo, but minimal other side effects. One day at a time (breathe), one day at a time (breathe), one day at a time – and this too shall be over!

# June 26

## Three Zaps Down

I have started my daily drive to New Richmond, Wisconsin, for radiation treatments. Three down, 30 to go. The first 25 are of the general area and final eight will be directed at the lump site. As the gals say at the clinic, what happens in that secured room appears to be "uneventful." I have counted the length of the two zaps I receive and have never gotten past 15 seconds for either. On the days I don't meet with the radiologist, I can be IN and OUT of the clinic doors in 15 minutes, which includes slipping off the upper clothing articles, putting on a big gown, getting settled into my own head/arm form, and redressing to leave.

Many medical treatments remind me of Star Trek... machines 'whirring' around making clicks and other sounds with invisible beams coming out. The expected side effects for radiation will be visible in the look of a 'sunburn' after a bit (I have medicated cream for that), along with the fatigue I have already mentioned. Apparently there is a need to consume more calories, especially protein, to assist with the body's reaction to 'fighting' what it senses as a foreign substance. I am grateful for summer days that will allow me the time needed to nap and 'hang-low.'

The past two days I was surprised at the quickness to which tears could erupt from my eyes. On one occasion, a woman stopped to talk in a Target store. I didn't know her name when we started our conversation. She is a three-year survivor who still faces challenges from her Stage IV diagnosis. Her total care, concern, and understanding of the disease immediately made her a part of my Breast Cancer's Bitchin' Club...and we had a teary meeting right there next to the doggie treats. I also became a puddle when the boys' pediatrician asked how I was doing. It seems whenever I "break" the news to someone I haven't seen in awhile, I can't keep it together. Yet other times, I can feel "matter of fact" about it all. Hormones are still going amuck. I just don't have any "cycle" to clock and keep track of as a 'warning' of stronger emotions! I will come up with a chemo acronym for PMS another time!

I've also been struggling with a fatigue I haven't had for awhile – I saw Dr. Williams for what turned out to be an outer ear infection (like swimmer's ear – only probably caused by sweat running down my head during heat waves while sleeping – heat incubating the bacteria – what else could it be?!) He did a check on my blood counts prior to the last big chemo. My last hemoglobin was 6.5 – normal is 12 – a bit lower is cause for a blood transfusion. He said getting that number back up could take months. (Huh? Not what I wanted to hear.) I grabbed some slow-release iron tabs to take, but need to wait until I am done with a new round of antibiotics.

We also talked about the pain in my upper right quadrant. I had already researched to learn it is an occasional message from my gall bladder. To be proactive, I am scheduled to have an ultrasound of the area to check for stones. Though I joked with Dr. Amy about this last 'useless' organ of mine, there's a chance we will see each other, again. It's the year of repairs and getting rid of unnecessary items! I've got a temporary cap on my tooth, too, with the real deal to be put in place after the 4th. I should have asked for gold.

With my cheaters and the sun shining on my legs earlier this week, I saw new hair! I decided I couldn't have 'peach fuzz' at the beach, so took after them with a razor in the shower. It's been 4 months since a blade has touched my skin! I keep checking my upper lip and chin for signs of growth – can't say I've been happy about appearance of hair in those areas in the past, but may do an 'alleluia' dance when it happens now. Psst...hear this in a whisper, "I've also got some prickly stuff coming in down below my bikini line." It's interesting how the loss was just a bit at a time, over weeks, and new growth appears to be coming back in the same fashion, in subtle patches. It's not like exposing yourself to the sun and getting an even tan. Now wouldn't it be something to step into an area with invisible rays of some type and presto – a full head of hair and evenly covered everywhere!

One story: It's the hour before bed once "curfew" at the lake has brought the boys inside our park model unit. The routine includes showers, snacks, and an attempt at getting them to read a bit before falling asleep. They use the bathroom in shifts, so as Matthias gets soaped up first, Tim and I stretch out on the love seat and couch, our heads resting on the ends near each other. He is tracking the words in a book as I read aloud. I've had it with my scarf and the heat, so take the bugger off. Tim doesn't mind, and for once, Matthias walks down the short hall towards us and doesn't make a big fuss about it.

He repeats what Tim has said the day before, "I can't remember what you look like with hair." And then he plops down on the little footstool next to me asking if he can touch "it." It's a tentative reach, while Tim quickly puts his hand on my head to reassure him, "It's not so bad."

Matthias gives a nervous chuckle as he places his on top adding, "Ewwww." I also feel the downy hair to say, "It's soft.' And though typical of these days, that Matthias and I can't agree, we all giggle and laugh during this time together.

You've got to take special moments as a counter to the yuck on a road trip like this, and Tim did confirm I have some darker little hairs growing "on top".

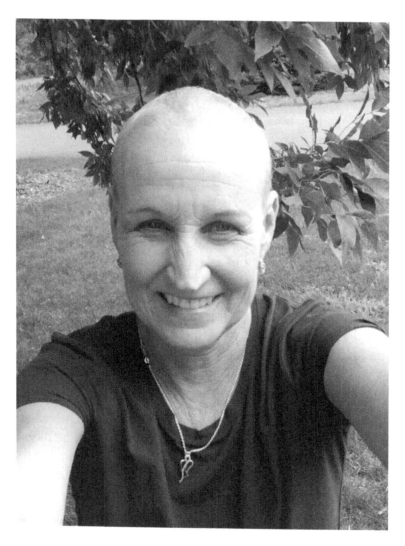

*The downy stuff.*

# July 11

## Five-Month Shadow

*"Good things come from a quiet place: study, prayer, music,
transformation, worship, communion. The words peace and quiet
are all but synonymous, and are often spoken in the same breath.
A quiet place is the think tank of the soul, the spawning ground
of truth and beauty... A quiet place outdoors has no physical
borders or limits to perception. One can commonly hear for miles
and listen even farther. A quiet place affords a sanctuary for the
soul, where the difference between right and wrong becomes more
readily apparent. It is a place to feel the love that connects all
things, large and small, human and not; a place where
the presence of a tree can be heard. A quiet place is
a place to open up all your senses and come alive."*

— Gordon Hempton

There are signs that I am moving toward recovering from chemo and tooth trauma. I know the saying usually refers to a guy's five o'clock shadow on the face, but I can boast I have a five-month shadow on my head! It's actually getting a little darker than the fine blond fuzz that hung on during my months of chemo treatments. I've heard numerous times, "It will come back thick and curly;

that's how a friend of a friend of a friend of my auntie's did." Actually, I had thick and wavy hair, so the few reports I've gotten about my normal kind was that it came back straight and fine. I have to say I never liked the way I looked during the 'perm' era, but will take what I get! It's kind of like the anticipated delivery of a baby; I wonder what it will look like?!

Yesterday, I had Taira out for what used to be my "short walk," as the goal for my new 'long walk,' instead of the 'not much of a walk' I have been doing. It felt great! On the return I marveled at the feeling of ENERGY coming back into my BEING. Geez, it's really been months since I have felt this way, and it was reassuring that the worst may actually be over. Radiation is said to cause fatigue as the days go by, but for now, I am savoring a sense of 'normalcy.' Today I walked her, again, without a hat. As we hit the gravel, Tim shouted out from his dirt bike to put one on. As I shook my head vigorously NO, he called out, "People know you. You will embarrass the family." Ha – little does he know, at 12, that embarrassing a family takes more than a walking down country roads with a chemo head!

Some of my family and friends have been "praying for the tooth." This week I am "chewing on the tooth" – a new crown, that is. The temporary 'cap' was on almost three weeks, so it's nice to use both sides of my molars to eat. I am a bit concerned about the extra wear and tear on "the other side." It's the aging thing. I also should make an eye appointment before school starts, too. The cheaters are moving up in magnification. Maybe I will consider contact lenses. Is that a sign of attempting to stay youthful?

Twelve of 33 radiation treatments done; the drive is more of a 'pain' than the zaps. (Sing along with me... "On the road, again. I don't wanna be on the road, again...") I made the trip from Webster three days last week. The boys were grateful to stay at the lake, and I enjoyed the company of one of my Mallard moms for one. We did a bit of thrift store shopping on the way back, while others kept tabs on our kids. The support continues as I move through this "not a journey," and it is much appreciated!

In talking with another 'radioactive' friend recently, we wondered about the 'radiation-god' who determines just what number will do the trick. In grumbling about the number deal, she shared that she was determined to get her 'certificate' upon completion. Though there really isn't one, it was something to put into my head in order to persevere these next weeks. "I am not a quitter, I am not a quitter, I am not a quitter"...that chant is needed, too! There is an incredible amount of faith one needs to put in modern medicine, but some days can leave you a doubter about human contraptions!

Others shared that the every-three-week Herceptin infusions didn't bother them, but I am dealing with some tingling in my fingers and sensitivity on the bottom of my feet, again. I had a dose yesterday. Of course, I am hoping it is just a "fluke" and not a side effect of the Herceptin. The neuropathy was appearing to be subsiding, but it's one day at a time, one treatment at a time, so I won't make any judgment calls on it, yet.

My nails continue to peel away. They are so short I can't even pick up a penny. I had to ask Tony to get a little dead tick off of Taira, because I couldn't get a-hold of it. I haven't had fingernails this stubby since biting them in my younger years and had forgotten how useful they can be! It's a bit frustrating. I didn't realize I used the side of my thumbnails to text, so I fumble with that lately, as well.

I have also purchased an "itty-bitty-bitta" to use in the bunk house. For those of you unfamiliar with the stories of the nine "Swedish-sisters," my mom and eight sisters shared a "bitta" in the hallway at night...it is what the English would call a "chamber pot." I found a cute one at Goodwill – though it doesn't have a cover. I won't need anyone "warming" it up for me before its use, though. Summer nights do that just fine. (Winter nights in Wisconsin presented a different situation for the Amys gals.)

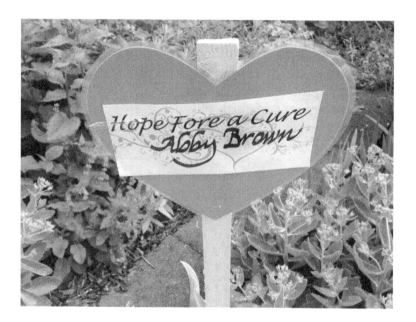

# July 25
## *Getting Felt Up There!*

I often find my hands checking out the new growth of hair on my head. I have moved into the stage of being 'felt-up-there' by others, as well. It started with the boys at home. Matthias, who has always been tentative about my baldness, is a head taller than me. The other day we stood next to each other in the bathroom at the lake. He has a good view from above and wanted to visually measure the ¼ inch accumulation lying on my head. He asked if it hurt as he pulled a tuft up. I think he was afraid if he tugged too hard, he would pull it out; heaven forbid! Tim and Tony have done their inspections, too, but it's also friends and 'strangers' who can't resist reaching to touch and commenting how 'soft' it is...like a baby chick. (I am still working on being a 'chick' but a baby I am not!)

My hands also check for breast tenderness, which is resulting from the radiation; they are needed to apply ointment to treat the skin-burn that is occurring there. That body part is left untouched by others, thank God, though Tony is privy. I will say it is nice to hear the excited comments about this sign of recovery. Add eye/eyebrow liner with a smile, and I do feel better!

Hair is growing elsewhere, too. There used to be tweezers in a compartment near my steering wheel in the van. Lately, while I drive, I have been using my stubby thumbnail and finger to pull out the new bristles I've discovered on my chin and upper lip. My belly and back feel bumpy, a bit like a rash, but it is prickly little hairs. When I wear my cheaters, I can see them on my arms, too. Yee-haw! Another sign of healing is visible in my fingernails. Though they are short, they seem to be toughening up, with potential to grow out, rather than peeling easily away.

Twenty-two of radiation treatments completed – I am 2/3 done! More days than I had planned, I have been continuing to make the drive from Mallard Lake to New Richmond, but being at the lake makes summer feel "more normal", and is a place for better relaxation. If I feel social, there is instant companionship with friends, but it also allows the alone time I need. The boys have a gaggle of kids to hang with, too. While there, I think we all forget, a little, about the cancer I have been dealing with for the last six months.

In looking ahead, I feel a special excitement about the start of the school year with my fifth and sixth graders. Being back in my classroom of 25 years, in the small community I love, will also return me to a state of normalcy.

For now, my bed-head in the morning is also tended to and quickly smoothed down by my hands. It will be interesting to see how my cowlicks spring up. I may need to add some spit before rubbing. The neuropathy has caused stiffness in the joints. I look like Grandpa McCoy (The Real McCoys – for those of you old enough to picture him hobbling) when I get up after sitting/driving, but time will take care of that. And one day at a time, it is!

# August 6

*Battered Boob, Hairy Knuckles*

It's amazing how an invisible 'ray' can make my breast feel as if someone has taken a rubber mallet to it. The nurse explained it's like a bruise without the color; the cells have been damaged and are healing. Bam, bam! Three *more* and I *graduate*! I guess there is some little ceremony from the staff at the end of these sessions, so I may get a certificate after all; I will find out on Friday!

The techs *et al* at New Richmond have been a delight to see weekdays for the last six weeks. Okay – not a delight, but they have been very pleasant. My 'chipper attitude' at being almost done caused an amused smile on the face of the radiologist on Monday. It was a drastic change from our first appointment when Tony handed me tissues, and I acted like a little kid. "I don't want to do this, and you can't make me! Explain why I should!" I think he wasn't sure if I would walk back through the doors after that meeting.

The techs chat as they get the machine all set up, proudly positioning it to the nearest millimeter. One exits the room with a little bounce to her step and a sing-songy, "Here we go!" One day I suddenly thought, *"No, there you go, and here I lie!"* In case you don't know, as they leave, there is a steel door that closes off the rest of the building from any radioactive material.

On another day, a side arm on the table was left out a bit on my right side. As the machine rotated above me for the next zap from this angle, it bumped into it. It stopped and bounced a bit as I let out a startled sound. In a split second my mind raced. "How do I take cover? Okay – breathe. You can roll to your left side, and onto the floor before the laser beam starts. It doesn't matter if your gown is still on the table and you are discovered huddled underneath, exposed from the waist up."

"We'll be right in," I hear simultaneously from the speaker in the ceiling, so I remained still in my position on top, with arms still overhead. "Don't shoot!" could have been an added thought here!

Though the boys continue to marvel at the growth of my head hair. I excitedly showed Matthias my little eyelashes this weekend. His comment, "Yah, big deal. At least you didn't have to worry about nose hair before." Really? Must be a guy thing! Tim and I compared his straight, dark leg hair to my stuff on top. I do have some 'blond' mixed in (maybe gray, too), but so far it is also stick straight. This is a change. When I sent a phone pic to my Mom, she replied, "Very interesting." When we talked, she did say she is happy about whatever it may be, and simply wants me to be healthy again.

I had to take a picture of my knuckle hair. It was an exciting discovery for me. I realize there are some who lose body hair that never returns. I don't mean to be over-exuberant about something so small, but in my case, it does indicate healthier days ahead. I do have a widow's peak that looks a bit like Eddie Munster combined with the Demi Moore look. You can call me G.I. Abby Munster.

Watch for one of my next posts when I share a story about the new hair-growth experienced by my friend, Toni-from-the-Marine-Garage... Back in the day, drugs used to kill her cancer cells were given in 'experimental' doses – stronger than my dose. I will have to rephrase it, though, to make it PG-13.

# August 8

## *Angels with Sue*

T he first member of my Breast Cancer's Bitchin' Club was Sue. She told me that many good things had come from her treatment...one being that she was no longer allergic to cats. She shared an upbeat attitude about her reality; she lives with cancer and had made peace with it. It wasn't robbing her of quality days. Sue taught band and shared her love of music with students in the Stillwater Area School District for years. She spent many of them with us at Marine Elementary including when she was first diagnosed. She was awe-inspiring as she stood before the students at the spring concert with her hat and smaller appearance. Her smile filled the room. The kids adored her.

When Sue was diagnosed with breast cancer on August 14, 2009, it had already moved to the liver and lymph nodes. She has 'fought the good fight,' as we are told to do, but is now receiving hospice care at home. She is surrounded with family and friends in these final days.

Needless to say, I understand this disease from an inside perspective, and an outside-looking in perspective. Cancer hurts. It breaks hearts.

The following is from Sue's Caring Bridge, posted today by a dear friend.

*Even here, in a living room centered by Sue in a hospital bed, and even now, when she is largely unable to respond to us who surround her, music is at the heart of this day.*

*Aunt Marlene, Pat, Craig, Barb, and I (Donna) are here, doing our best to keep Sue comfortable and to keep her feeling our devotion. We know that others are coming soon and/or staying with her in their thoughts and spirits. She feels you, too.*

*My favorite moment of the day (so far):*

*I brought a couple of Lake Wobegon Brass Band CDs, and as they played, I was narrating them to her. "Here's Sue, playing the snare drum and looking at Donna on the cymbals, telling her with her eyes not to come in yet!" She would let out a small grin or open an eye, showing that she was hearing and comprehending.*

*Then, when "The Little Drummer Boy" came on, she sat up – well, popped up, really. She held Barb's hands in front of her, while Craig held one arm and I held the other. There we were, a "circle of love" for the entire song. It was amazing.*

*Now, the show tunes are serenading us as she rests with the help of some gentle painkillers and her dad holding her hand.*

*So, turn on your favorite music and listen to it. It would make Sue happy to know that you are enjoying her true passion.*

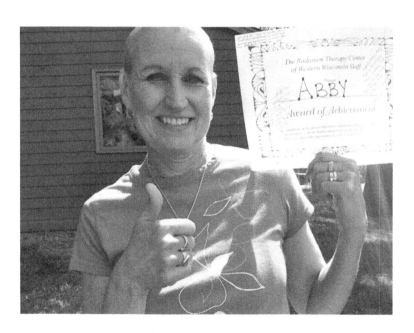

*Certifiably done with radiation!*

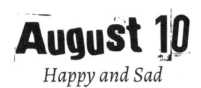
# August 10
## *Happy and Sad*

Yesterday was my official graduation from radiation. I really *did* get a certificate – for the 33 treatments; It is now hanging on the refrigerator along with one that recognizes my 25 years with the Stillwater School District.

These treatments are called zingers – from the inside out. One of my BCBC friends said her skin was actually black from her radiation treatment – (yikes.) Poison and burns are the prescribed regimen for becoming a cancer survivor. I was told to expect fatigue to continue for another week or more. Apparently, my skin fared better than others...it doesn't look much worse than a sun burn, though my pain is similar to others due to the damage of the nerve tissue and cells. After all of this, I'd rather call myself a Treatment Survivor.

The cancerous mass has been gone since my lumpectomy in January; the chemo/radiation regimen certainly took care of anything microscopic. I'm done with the "tough" stuff. Tamoxifen pills for five years and Herceptin infusions every three weeks until next May will be the easier part of this.

My excitement over the completion of the radiation is tempered by the loss of Sue Moran yesterday afternoon. This disease continually has hearts aching. She will be missed on earth.

There is no humor for today's post. We need to take the good with the bad, one day at a time. Love and hugs to all.

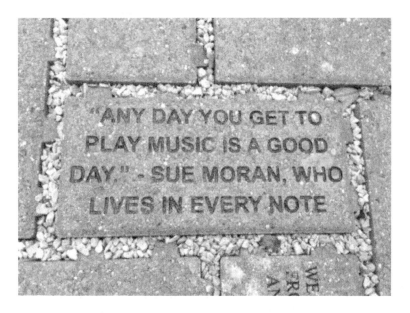

*Susan Anne Moran, December 15, 1966 – August 9, 2013, Age 46.*

# August 14
## *Time Away*

I have only one appointment in these last two weeks of 'summer vacation.' I scheduled time away with a couple of girlfriends. Slot tournament, chatter, movies, time on a pontoon...that kind of get away! You know the kind that make your stomach hurt and potentially cause a leak from the bladder? (Not mine, my boys were adopted; I wore my jeans home from the hospital after their births. *Wink.*) We had a delightful time and captured many silly moments on camera ("don't ask" type shots). Fun!

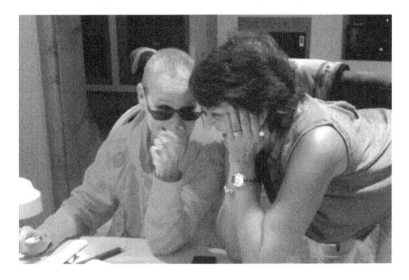

*Giggling gals – thanks, Robin!*

My breast tissue continues to be tender. I have not been pushing the activity, yet, though we did take a good walk together. The days are just ahead for getting my muscles back in shape!

# August 19

*UTI? Nooo! Yep.*

Today was the first day I hadn't taken anything to deal with potential pain due to the radiation and neuropathy. So, when I realized, this afternoon, that I could have a "bladder and parts" infection, it was with full-nerve sensations. (Yikes!)

In my 54 years, I've never had one, and I now know how lucky I have been! Good God, they are painful. When the urgent care doctor confirmed my lab results he added, "Yes, your white count is very high. You've got a roaring infection." And he didn't even hear me in the bathroom sounding like a lion when I peed! (Grrrrr!)

This doctor continued to educate me. Apparently, the number one factor that impacts this type of infection for women is not emptying the bladder after sex. Really? I didn't know this, and shared that I've been married for 31 years and have never had this problem. I always head to the bathroom when the fireworks are over...and even sit patiently to wait for things to flow. (Girls in a happy relationship will understand what I mean...if you don't, bring it up at your next book club meeting or ask an honest woman.)

To save the doc time, I updated him on my recent chemo/radiation treatments and didn't hesitate to say that my oncologist said to do whatever "felt good" in that department. It's not much, I informed him, so I suggested that though Tony and I did take care of long overdue business this weekend, maybe I was out of practice. He wasn't familiar with my attempts at humor to deal with my recent illness, so was caught off guard by my remark. Of course he laughed. Really, what else can you do to balance the tears that accompany cancer?

Just so you know, this newest reason for a trip to the clinic could also be from riding a bike this weekend or being too lazy to get out of bed this morning when I got the first signals my bladder was full. Getting up would have meant the start of my last Monday morning at the lake, and though I am thrilled I will be back in the classroom, summer has gone by too quickly, again.

I am now taking two types of pills; (one that will turn the toilet water orange), I was told. I was grateful for the warning; the blood present in my urine today already had me alarmed. Since I've never had one of these, I didn't know it could also be a symptom. I sat in the waiting room talking to my heavenly friends. "Please don't send me to ER or for an overnight stay at Lakeview...we are suppose to be done with this... I start school in one week... I want to close this book." Requests granted. The doc told me I should be feeling better within 24 hours, and then this too will pass. Wow! I haven't had a 24-hour cure for *anything* over the last year.

Our family had a wonderful weekend at Mallard Lake, together. The highlight for me was an event that had many of us "kicking the asphalt" – four miles around the lake. I made it! And it felt great! The generous donations of this special group of people significantly impacted Cassie's fundraising efforts for the Three-Day Walk coming up this weekend. Both she and Anne met their goals by today's deadline. I am so blessed by the endless support of family and friends. It truly felt like a celebration of *the end* of the icky chemo and radiation treatments.

This morning, Matthias told me I had "real hair" and commented I should keep it short like this. I guess that means he likes it! Hats to be worn only because I want to from now on!

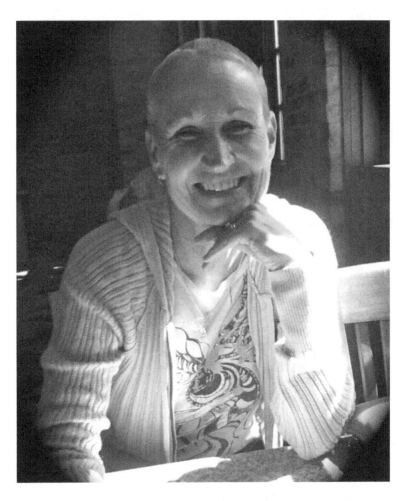

*August sunshine.*

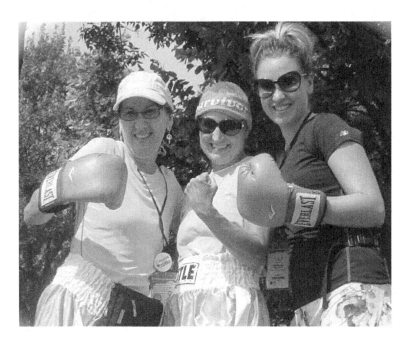

*Kickin' it – my sister, Anne, and my niece, Cassie, doing 60 miles.*

# August 25

*Looking in the Rearview Mirror*

When I was first diagnosed with breast cancer, I spent much time in conversation with a friend who had just finished up with final 'touches' from a bilateral mastectomy. We shared tears, and she passed on encouragement: "Before you know it, you will be looking in the rearview mirror, and this will all be behind you."

Along the way, my sister and niece decided to participate in the Susan G. Komen in my honor. At the time, the event, scheduled in August, seemed so far away. This afternoon, I stood on the Minnesota State Capitol grounds during the closing ceremony of the Three-Day Walk. Cassie and Anne were with 1,000 who walked in the heat these past days. They were surround by an additional thousand who supported their efforts on behalf of research, detection, treatment, and care of men and women in our country who battle this disease. It was an emotional day for me.

Despite a diagnosis and months of treatment, I still feel like cancer is something that happens to other people. It seems unreal to me that I now belong to an exclusive club and have an instant bond with the members I meet every day. Unfortunately, these days it is not a road less traveled. There are many of us. It's not a journey; it's a bumpy road trip.

Tomorrow I return to the classroom. Where has the time gone? Living in the moment can be a magic charm for getting through even the most unbearable of life's challenges. It's with faith that I have learned worrying about the future is not an effective use of energy.

Cancer is hard on families, too. But today, as my mom and I hugged and sobbed on the Capitol grounds, at least I could say, "It's over. We are done with this."

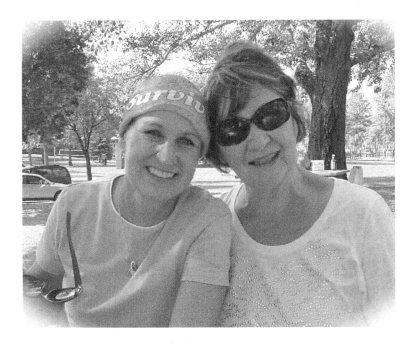

*A mother's love.*

# September 14

## *The Final Chapters*

It has been almost ten years since I seriously decided to tackle another disease. Alcohol no longer is a part of my diet. During the early stages of that first recovery, I'd have drinking dreams. It was always a relief to wake up to realize the worries of my sleep had not actually occurred.

Last night I had a very parallel "cancer biopsy" dream. Friends in my 'club' have mentioned that they are nervous before their annual check-ups. I've said that I didn't think this would bother me. But maybe I am wrong. In my dream the nurse was taking samples from the back of my neck. It didn't hurt – I was being tough. The thoughts of some kind of cancer metastasizing elsewhere in my body were a part of this nocturnal experience. I was taking it in stride, though.

People have asked me, "When do you get checked so you know the cancer's gone?" When I visited the radiologist this past week he said, "Come back in a year. I will leave the mammogram schedule up to your oncologist, Dr. Corey."

When my lump was removed on January 22, I considered myself cancer free. Previous tests showed no others signs of cancer in either breasts or my bones. The one lymph node removed was clean, and Dr. Fox removed a good margin around the tumor. The chemo was a "safety" precaution. I don't have any plans to do the "hard-stuff" again.

The disease of alcoholism has its challenges, and with faith, strength, hope, and support of others for self-control, the bottle can be eluded. But cancer plays on a different field. Most of us with cancer didn't do anything specific to cause the disease to progress. So in comparison, cancer feels out of my control. And with that said, I have to put it into the hands of my faith partners, those on earth and those above. Though my dream hinted at fear, in reality my path will still be taken one step at a time, through each day, with confidence that I can meet the challenges that come along the way.

For today, I deal with the neuropathy flaring up after the tri-weekly infusions of Herceptin (these will continue until May 2014.) I hadn't expected it, but it is what it is. Soon, I will start an oral-type chemo to take for five years. And I've read that post-treatment depression can occur, but my time with kids in the classroom and caring for two dogs and family each evening doesn't leave much room for spending thoughts on cancer. Yep, two dogs. We are now foster parents for Gus, my niece's English Lab, as she ventures off to Ecuador to teach English to high schoolers. (Both are sweethearts!)

If tears come, they are necessary, but to the greater extent, all is right in my world. My breast is still tender, but healing. And yep, it is a bit smaller and perkier than the other one, but I have no intentions of participating in any reconstructive procedure to "reduce and lift" for a match. "Tough titties" to both of them!

My prayer: May the ascended masters of history and the powers that lead us bring growth and a vision toward our purpose and mission on Earth – you, me, and that of our loved ones. May your spirits shine! Thank you for being a part of my life's travels. Much love to all.

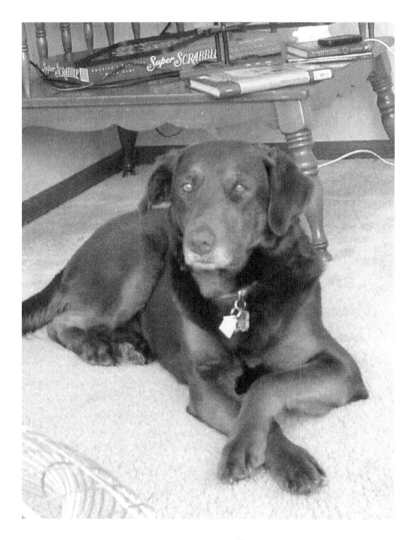

*A pose to remember.*

# October 7

## *For the Love of Dogs*

"Taira! Come, Taira! Come on. Good girl..." That is my usual call when I have both dogs out for a walk in our back acreage. We live on six and a half, technically, but the three of us always use the mowed paths that wrap around the sides and behind our property.

That doesn't mean Gus and Taira stay on the trail. They both romp in and out of the sumac brush, sniffing and running. They chase each other, and Gus will run ahead and circle-back several times bounding with joy. I laugh at them, relishing the reason to be outside, smelling the grass and listening to the sound of the birds wind through the trees.

During these giddily roam about, their tongues hang out of their mouths; I can hear the panting, even when I can't see them. I also hear the jingle of the name and rabies tags on their collars. But sometimes Taira goes out of earshot. And it makes me a little nervous. She isn't the best about coming when called, especially if she gets a whiff of something other critter's trail. But on a recent backyard adventure, she noticed another dog and its owner walking along the road in front of our house.

It was a dog owner's nightmare. She'd been gone a bit, despite my calls. We were mid-way back when I'd lost sight and sound of her. I called for Gus, who appeared in his usual manner. I continued my usual chant, "Taira! Come on! Good girl!"

And then the alarming sounds came. I heard the barking, high pitch yelps, and the voice of a woman screaming. My heart raced, and I started to run toward the commotion. As I came over the hill, I spotted Taira. She was standing next to a woman yelling and waving her arms frantically. I recognized her and knew her older female Golden Retriever did not take well to other dogs.

Panic set in as my mind raced, along with my legs. I had to get to them, but couldn't do it fast enough. My calls to Taira become frantic, but I also had Gus and needed to get him back to the house before getting to her.

"Get! Go away! Bad dog!" are the words coming from the road.

"She's not!" my mind shouts back.

Gus was trained by my niece and brother-in-law as a pup. Thank goodness he listens well and followed me into the house as I grabbed the keys to the van. When I arrived to break up the dog-tussle, I was able to get Taira into our vehicle on the opposite side of the road, but in my distress, I didn't close the door. Her collar had fallen off, and the woman shook it at me, understandably upset and shouting, "I hope she's had her rabies shots."

As I began to apologize and reply, "Yes," Taira charged out of the van door and right back at the dog.

"Stop it! Stop it, bad dog!" sounded again.

It took all my muscle to lift Taira up and off the Golden Retriever she had pinned to the ground. I rolled her away. We both had hearts beating rapidly as I sat with my legs wrapped around her in the middle of that dirt road. But mine began to ache. I knew that though she did her best to protect me, I couldn't protect her from the possible decisions humans would make about her place in our world.

After quickly getting Taira back to the house, I returned to the Retriever and her owner, driving them home with a true concern for the this dog. I know what it's like to love them, and completely understood her worries, though mine were now of a different nature. She also understood that I was equally upset by the situation.

When I arrived back home to the garage, Taira greeted me with her tail wagging. My heart sunk as I petted her, and with tears in my eyes I started the process of obtaining advice from MN PAWS. The days that followed would be unbelievably difficult.

# October 19

## *Angels Sent Her*

It is only recently that I have given the news to Matthias and Tim that Taira didn't go to another home. Although it was an extremely difficult decision, staff from MN PAWS felt that looking for new owners couldn't be done in good faith. She had a 'history' of dog-aggression before she came to us, and we experienced another incident at the lake this summer. Everyone agreed that she was a people lover. But her life prior to arrival in Minnesota made her a risk to other dogs and their owners. As the caring vet gave the injection, she rested in my lap on the floor. It took bravery I didn't know I possessed to be with her. She was 'my girl.' Tears flow quickly as I think of her.

She brought joy to all of us during this challenge and gave the boys someone to talk to when "Mom" was sick. There was something heartwarming about seeing our 14-year-old scratch her behind the ears, while looking into her eyes to chat. "You're a good girl, Taira. Yah, you're a good girl," he'd coo-coo at her. She allowed them to show their gentle, softer sides. Thank goodness we have Gus to still provide this for the boys.

Life is filled with love and loss. But faith puts her spirit by my side. She sent a sign through Gus that she is alright. He placed his paw onto my forearm yesterday, in the same fashion Taira always did. It's not something he had ever done before. My Mom texted me a message, "Angels sent Taira to you." And in a symbolic way, I see her absence in our lives as a sign that so is the cancer.

I miss her.

Despite the ups and downs, my days continue with the 'usual' school routine and boys at home. As I move forward out of the cancer treatment days, I am reminded there is always something for somebody to face and grow through while we spend time on Earth. So many such things have happened recently.

I have sent prayers to angels for the newest member of my school's family. She has spent her first month in neonatal ICU due to a traumatic birth – yet her parents speak words of incredible faith. Their daughter is slowing healing, miraculously maybe, but not surprisingly, if you believe in the powers above.

My BCBC buddy, Toni, always gave me daily encouragement to get through the tough days. She now mourns the loss of her father-in-law, who died tragically in a car accident at 80 years old recently. He was a much-loved man in our community, and his death leaves many struggling with his absence.

Also, my sister has been dealing with the theft of several thousand dollars from their bedroom. She and Mark are selling and building, and her hidden stash of eight years was unconsciously moved to a more conspicuous spot in transition and disappeared during a house showing or photo shoot for advertising their river home. One could consider it "just money," but it's unsettling. She is an incredible giver of time and gifts and a real angel on earth as we say.

And our oldest deals with the questions of an adolescent uncertain of his future. "What if I'm not successful in life, Mom?" As we lie on his bed in the dark, it's the 'faith' part of my reassurance that I hope he absorbs into his being. It's the only way I know people come through, and over time, heal from challenges. It is certainly what has gotten me through this cancer battle.

Yesterday, I was unpacking hats from the lake – the ones my aunties made me and others I wore before my hair started to sprout. We are on a two-day break. I had three days with students and two full nights of conferences earlier this week. I was tired and had a minute to think... My eyes began to brim with tears as my mind delved back into memories of the last nine months. And then it came to me again, I want this to be over. I don't want to continue the Herceptin every-three-weeks until May. But am I brave enough to say, "NO MORE. I've done enough"? I am now struggling with that. My feet throb and ache, my knees and fingers are stiff. How much more do I endure to guarantee I have an even smaller chance of recurrence in the years ahead? (There are no guarantees.)

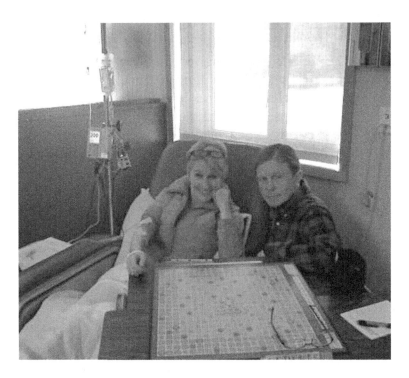

*Back to that first day.*

# October 23

## *A Little Trim*

**M**y hair was getting shaggy. For real. Today I had a little trim – a bit off the neckline and some evening-out of the straggly ends. I think it looks a tad bit better. That's all I can say about it – short and simple.

I had another Herceptin infusion yesterday. I've been online, reading research on the protocol of these infusions. They are only for HER2 positive patients. My prescribed regimen is to continue every three weeks until May. I have had 15 Herceptin infusions since April, and according to some, that is enough.

"With cost-effectiveness and patient convenience in mind, there is a lot of attention on how long to give this drug," breast cancer specialist Dr. Edith Perez of the Mayo Clinic says "It may be that two years is better than one, but it may also be that three months is better than two years."

The estimated cost for one year of Herceptin is about $50,000 a year, and one research project confirmed that two years had the same results as one year. There are additional research studies looking at the impact of nine-week and six-month treatment plans. And some countries with a taxpayer-funded public health system, such as New Zealand, have opted to fund only nine weeks of therapy as a result of research that indicated nine weeks was as effective as a year.

It is reassuring that I have done plenty to tackle any possible cancer cells that were in my body last January. At the time of my lumpectomy, there were no visible signs of any kind, anywhere else, so this may really be the beginning of my cancer's end.

It's uncanny how complacency can set into the thinking of a cancer patient and family after months of chemo sessions. There have been times I needed to remind myself, and the boys, that I don't feel well, because I JUST HAD CHEMO. "Oh, yah, chemo again...big deal..." I have to admit I forgot to "close the lid and flush twice" last night.

But earlier in the day I watched a "newbie" prepping for her first infusion. It *is* a big deal, and my emotions became raw as I heard the nurse go over chemo effects on blood cell counts, what to do in case of fever, and so on. Her husband listened and watched his wife with the look of love laced with worry and concern. She was nodding her head in what I know was a fogged understanding as his eyes filled with tears. She was being brave.

It took me back to my first day in that chair and I wanted to take it away for her, from both of them. The emotions swelled up in my chest and out. I didn't even know her, but felt protective and cried for the days ahead. Days she doesn't understand at this time. Days I don't wish on anyone.

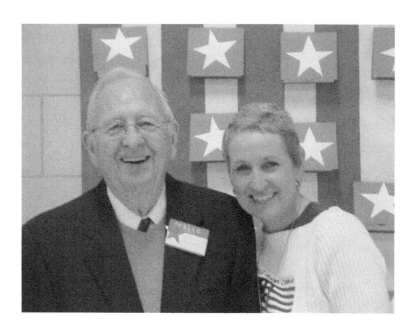

*Dad and I.*

# November 11

## A Day of Reflection

It can be tough to make decisions about the different types of challenges we face. They have to be based on what choices we have at the time, and for me decision-making is a mix of faith, intuition, and current medical facts. I have another Herceptin infusion scheduled this week; I made the appointment today. Tony and I will visit with Dr. Corey, my oncologist, later next week.

Questioning the medical 'prescription' isn't what others would do. I can't say why I feel I have a choice to make, but it's there in my heart. You can be certain, I have had my share of 'you can't quit now' words of encouragement from those who care about me. So, it goes back to one day at a time. For this one, no final decision has been made about the next recommended seven more months of infusions...

All families deal with tough stuff. Besides this cancer road trip I've been on, my family has also been struggling with the question of how to best care for aging parents. My dad was diagnosed with dementia six years back, and we are starting to feel that part of him is slowly being taken away from us.

Yesterday, Dad and I spent time going through a box of newspaper clippings, photos, and additional keepsakes from his younger years. He wrapped himself in these days from the past as best he could. I found his original enlistment papers and assignment to serve with the United States Air Force as a dentist during the Korean War from 1953-55. He went directly from his graduation out of dental school at Marquette, WI, as a 24-year-old man.

Today (Veteran's Day), he joined other veterans at our little elementary school for a special assembly honoring them. As the children sang patriotic songs, emotions came forth from vets and family members alike. I knew enough to load my pockets with tissues for this time of remembering and reflecting.

For me, my dad isn't just to be honored for service for his country, but for the countless ways in which he contributed toward the good in our world. His love for his family and friends still emanates through his being. In spite of any daily confusion he exhibits, he continues to be clear about a God above and a place for each of us in heaven. God bless his soul on Earth.

I love you, Dad.

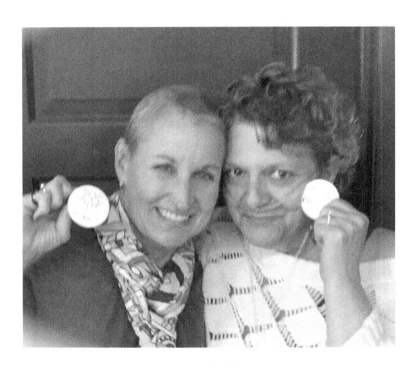

*Bosom buddies.*

# November 17

## *Precious Fighters*

As Matthias sat behind me in the car one day, he commented that I needed to shave. I thought he meant my lip hair, but he clarified I had a beard. He was right. It reminded me of a story Toni-from-the-Marine-Garage told me.

When Toni was first diagnosed with breast cancer over 13 years ago, she was part of research studies for many of the chemo drugs approved and used as common infusions today. The difference was in the potency. She says the stuff about killed her.

She warned me of the 'baby' growth of hair that would come first...like that on newborns – all over the body. It's soft and fine, and what Matthias noticed on my cheeks was blond. When I had my first 'trim' this fall, my stylist took a razor to it. It hasn't grown back, unlike the lip hair that he still reminds me needs 'shaving.'

Toni's complexion and hair are darker than mine. When she first noticed the growth on her face, she said it looked like that of a guy's. In a frantic mode, she called her oncologist. "What did you do to me?! When I agreed to this, you didn't tell me it would increase my testosterone! I look like a man!

What should I expect next?! A 'thing' to sprout between my legs?!" If you know Toni, you know she didn't use the word "thing" when ranting and raving to her doctor. Replace it with any four letter word used to describe that particular male body part, and you've got the Toni version.

As I have said before, chemo patients feel like guinea pigs at times. We share stories of understanding with each other that family and friends don't quite get. We know you do your best to listen and learn, though. The empathy you give to us on this bumpy road trip is always appreciated.

Toni continues to live with cancer and volunteers to experiment with new chemo drugs. She is *precious* to all.

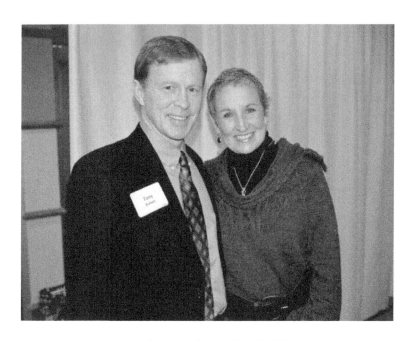

*In sickness and returning health.*

# November 24

*How Big is Your Brave?*

This past week I had the opportunity to speak at the Lakeview Health Foundation's community breakfast. In preparing, the foundation director and I chatted about a theme. There are many songs out there that emphasize being brave. One that struck home to me, though, is one sung by Josh Groban. It's not about being brave for oneself. "My reason to be brave" is for others. When cancer patients are told they are "being brave" in the face of a diagnosis, I'd bet that most go through treatment for the sake of those they love on earth. It's an integral part of what we do.

In the twelve minutes allocated for me to speak, in front a nice group of about 250, I shared past journal entries that highlighted my experiences with our local community hospital, clinic, and health care providers. It made the audience laugh and cry. And the feedback afterwards was affirming. My story isn't much different than other cancer patients, but writing about it with a little honesty and grit has been appreciated by many. It speaks for those impacted by the diagnosis, I've been told. And it educates others.

I've been encouraged to turn my writing into a book. Taking time to seek out appropriate advice, a potential editor, and a publishing company hasn't gone in my favor. But as it can go in the life of someone who has faith, it is all coming together. One of the students in my first class at Marine Elementary, a 5th grader at the time, contacted me. Kent is now older than I was when I was his teacher 25 years ago. He is a motivational coach, author, founder of Blooming Twig, and we have used modern communication to begin the process of putting this story together.

It's an experience linked to purpose – my reason to be brave.

"You wanna run away, run away,
And you say that it can't be so,
You wanna look away, look away,
But you stay, because it's all so close,
When you stand up and hold out your hand,
In the face of what I don't understand,
My reason to be brave!"

— Josh Groban

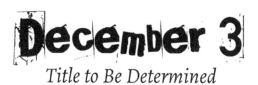

# December 3

## *Title to Be Determined*

I finally got started editing my journal entries this past week. I am a procrastinator by nature (thanks, Dad) but realized I was a bit afraid to take myself 'back there' to the beginning of this road trip. I have to say I was proud of myself for getting started. It seemed to be going quite well.

When the snow fell today, I took a minute to watch it outside my classroom window and reflect. My students had left the room to attend music class. We're working on knitting hats for premies and siblings at a local intensive care unit for a community service winter project. I was thinking about Toni-from-the-Marine-Garage, hoping she is doing okay, and suddenly, "whoosh." I was overcome with emotions. The snow and hats and thoughts of scarves to keep my bare head warm... Has it really been almost a year since my breast cancer diagnosis? Will I associate it with winter from now on? It was long and hard – I want to forget it, but it's still too raw.

I still find myself caught off-guard when I look in the mirror. I feel like ME on this inside. Our beings are so much more than the physical body. My mom and I talked about this awhile back...how aging doesn't seem to make you feel like a different YOU. It does allow for a more mature, wiser, patient being, but there's still sameness in the essence of our SOUL. Sometimes, it can be hard to grasp this concept with a true universal understanding. But for me, I find comfort in believing there is something greater. I need to remind myself that human emotion and tears are okay. (I'll be fine!)

It is still a wonder, though, as I reread and continue to write about a road trip I didn't want to take – did this really happen to me?

It's like dirty laundry. Life's challenges are unavoidable. Thank goodness for opportunities to immerse in soap and water. Sometimes coming out clean takes getting jostled around, but we can emerge to dry-out and take on the next mud pile.

(It's better than getting stuffed in a drawer, unchallenged, unworn.)

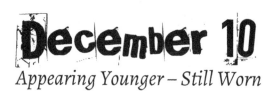

# December 10

*Appearing Younger – Still Worn*

I recently asked my boys how they felt when they learned about my cancer diagnosis. "I knew you wouldn't die," said Tim.

Matthias stated it more positively, "I knew you'd survive."

It's reassuring to hear that my months of treatment didn't leave them scarred in anyway. In contrast, I'd like to think that it made them stronger in some way.

This week, both made it clear that my new head of hair wasn't to their liking. Matthias hadn't done a "head-rub" for a while. As we sat together on the couch talking, he did a gentle lift of a tuft and exclaimed, "Whoa, you've got two inches here," and then showed me a measurement between his thumb and forefinger. This, before announcing that the color was bugging him. "You look old."

Tim quantified it, "Your hair makes you look 75."

Okay. Point taken. It's been described as "silver" by some, and Tony told the boys, if I were a horse, it would be called 'dapple gray." A horse I'm not, and an old-looking mother I didn't want to be, so my stylist fixed me up a bit today.

During a recent chat with my friend, Toni, she reminded me that if you didn't look older after cancer treatment, there's something wrong with you. I have to admit, I felt a little reluctant to give up one of my 'badges of courage.' Though the style is still short, it's not as obvious that I have undergone the 'horrors of chemo.' Which reminded me that there are many men and women who have endured the same, but at some point, you can't tell when you meet them on the street.

In time, we all have hidden battle scars. Remember that. And as Ellen Degeneres says at the end of each program, "Be kind to one another."

# December 25

## *A Cancer Road Trip in Video*

This is a small gift for you, family and friends, old and new. I love you.

Into the New Year, one day at a time, with angels watching over all!

Watch here:

https://www.YouTube.com/watch?v=N__xZ3mnPiw

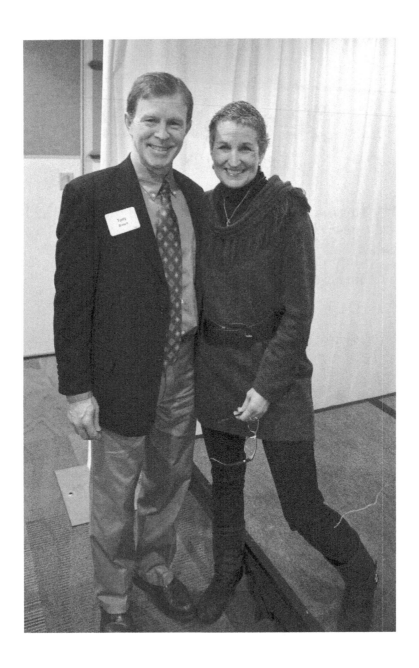

# December 31

*Back Together Again & Love's Endurance*

B ack together again...sharing the same bed, that is. Except that I just caught a bug, so coughing became an issue at night. That's always been one reason why Tony and I have slept in separate rooms. It certainly isn't due to lack of love for each other. If he is snoring (or I am) we know there is an extra bunk bed to crawl into for a good night's sleep; we don't take it personally.

When we were first married, I decided to head out to Pennsylvania to be a director of a summer Weight Watcher's camp for girls. It was a professional decision; one that Tony supported. It had us apart for almost 2 months. A couple years later, while substitute teaching in Steven's Point, Wisconsin, I learned that I enjoyed the elementary classroom setting. So I spent a semester living with Tony's folks to complete my Master's degree at the University of Wisconsin – La Crosse, adding elementary education to my license.

I likened our relationship to that of my parents. My mom had gone back to college when we were in elementary school to earn her business-education teaching certificate. To pay the tuition, she saved money from her 'allowance' and wallpapered for others. Dad honored her need for independence and a professional life. They each had their own social activities, but also spent much time together on vacations without my sisters and me. They also had countless dinners and dancing dates at the Elk's Club each week, while 'us girls' reveled in the overnights of doting by Grandma Shirley at her apartment.

Tony and I spent most nights together after my initial professional development, until the boys came along. I read-up on the benefits of sleeping with your children, and after years of waiting for them to arrive, we even did a family bed for a bit. As they grew, I learned to brush my teeth before laying down to read a bedtime story. As I scratched backs and sang lullabies, it was easy to fall asleep alongside one of them. I'd usually crawl into bed with Tony in the middle of the night, after my bathroom break, but not always.

Since our investment in a little Jayco 5th wheel, followed by our park-model little house at Mallard Lake Family Resort in Wisconsin, I still spend many summer weekdays with the boys 'at the lake', while Tony works and stays at home. And after he built the bunkhouse out back on our property, most of my summer nights at home are spent out there. Just so you know, that is after I tuck him into our bed inside... (couple-business taken care of first, as needed.)

I've learned he sleeps in the middle of our queen bed when he's going it solo. I don't. Just a silly observation.

Much of the past year, Tony slept down the hall, or downstairs when Tim moved upstairs. Our bedroom became my recovery room. My sleep schedule was different than his. He got up early to walk Taira, made breakfast for the boys, and then drove to work in Minneapolis. Some nights the steroids had me up late, but most mornings I woke up in time to kiss Tim goodbye and to wave at him from the living room window as the school bus pulled away.

My cancer treatment challenges are coming to an end. In addition to my video culmination, I had a photo of Tony and me made into a canvas portrait. It was taken after my presentation at the Lakeview Health Foundation breakfast – a highlight of my recovery. He teared up when he opened this gift. It symbolizes a real return to health.

My parents are entering the years where aging presents new challenges. My dad's dementia has progressed to a stage where we three daughters feel he cannot be left alone, just as if he is a little one in the toddler stage. And Mom doesn't get a good night's rest with his wandering patterns, so sleep deprivation is impacting her health. We are fortunate to have found a memory care unit just up the street from their townhome, an easy walk for her on a sunny, warm day. Dad is excited about his new 'place' and has even started his own "packing." She has spent days crying about the inevitable change for them.

When I was going through my treatment, she would often send messages that said, "I wish I could take this away for you." As we move into 2014, these are now my words to her. It is difficult to see her heart breaking, but it is with love and faith that I remind her, she can always "tuck him in" in his special bunk house and then move down the street for a good night's sleep. Angels will watch over them both, and their love for each other will endure.

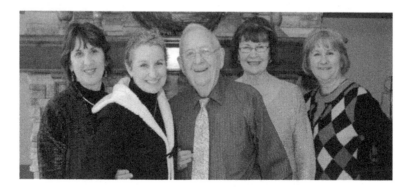

*The Marquarts: Anne, Abby, Art, Dianne, and Kristine.*

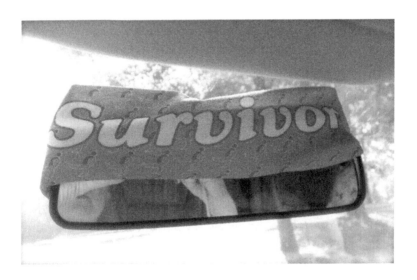

*Looking in the rear view mirror.*

# 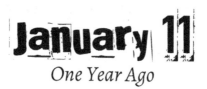 January 11

*One Year Ago*

I am feeling at a loss for words, but I have a need to write. It began when I learned that a friend from my BCBC group found a "new" lump. Her surgery was this past week; many cancerous lymph nodes were removed. This special friend was the one who shared, "Someday, you'll be looking in the rearview mirror at all of this." Gol' darn it, she is looking forward, again. (Dammit, really.)

We spent time talking together in her living room this afternoon. She didn't have chemo and radiation two years ago. It wasn't deemed necessary at the time, but it is now.

We only cried for a minute, then got to business by sharing information that breast cancer patients need from each other. It's a bitch, this breast cancer business.

I wish I didn't have a trunk full of hats and scarves to share with her. But I do. And I will teach her how to make a "sweet wrap" around her bare head.

It was one year ago, today, that Tony and I sat together to hear my official diagnosis. His birthday is on Monday. I will have a "one-year" mammogram done that afternoon, along with a bone density test to establish a baseline before beginning the prescribed five-year pills.

I am trying not to be nervous. It seems that goes with the road-trip, though. Note: I am still forgoing the use of the word 'journey' to describe all of this.

I hope my writing helps others, someday. For now, I'll consider the publishing of these words a real journey on which to embark!

# January 13
## *My True Love*

By the time it was confirmed that my lump was cancerous last January, I had a week to process the thought. I had started getting my "big girl attitude" in check, but struggled with breaking the news to my parents. Tony was the one to drive solo to their place and fill them in; my sisters happened to be visiting, so my diagnosis was delivered in one 'blow.'

Tony was by my side for all of the major infusions and surgeries physically and then in spirit as I was wheeled away to the sterile rooms. As the year went on, my independence was able to get me to daily radiation and the additional appointments that were required.

I intended to walk myself into imaging at Lakeview Hospital for my 'annual mammogram' this morning. When Tony asked what time the appointment was, I knew he wanted to come with me. After 31 years of marriage, words aren't always necessary to 'read' each other and know what the other one needs. I didn't want to make light of the significance of the procedure. Truthfully, I wanted to have him drive me to town, just as we had done so many times in the past year. Besides, it was his birthday. I suggested we have lunch together, after.

I have often mentioned that being strong is the only option most of us consider, yet our hearts ache for the pain we have unintentionally inflicted on our loved ones. I knew I was a bit edgy about my mammogram today. But I had done a good amount of squishing and palpating of my still-tender breast to feel confident there was nothing to be really worried about. We traveled to Stillwater in our usual silence, both lost in our own similar thoughts. For us, the year of "bad news" and treatment could make any appointment one that we expected to bring "more of the same" – especially given that I had extras thrown-in, with my appendix and mastitis. I didn't realize how difficult today would be for Tony, until I walked out of the dressing room.

The layout of the women's breast health rooms doesn't allow for male spouses to be present during the mammogram. They'd have to walk through the special waiting room ~ a quiet space with a fireplace and relaxing music that excludes guys. He was also told he couldn't be with me during the bone density x-ray, though this was no big deal. As the nurse announced my name for each procedure, Tony would start to gather his things to join me, then sit down with subtle signs of disappointment.

So he sat patiently reading in the imaging waiting room. We sat next to each other between the two tests, and I joined him in my half-gown (you can keep your pants on for these things, these days) after my parts were pulled, placed, and smashed between the two clear 'shelves.' We chatted about magazine articles while we waited to hear if there was to be a need for an follow-up ultrasound. It's what they do when there is something suspicious and a radiologist needs better images. (Been there, done that.)

Finally, the technician stuck her head out of the "women's room" looking for me. I guess I was supposed to stay in that one, rather than hang out with him in the waiting room meant for 'all-other' imaging appointments.

"You are going to get me in trouble!" I was told as I approached her.

Tony stood, attempting to inquire, again, if he could come with me. Nope. I watched him plop back down on the chair as she and I disappeared behind the door. So he waited some more.

The sun was shining through the waiting room window, at least. And it was quiet; people don't make loud conversation in clinics or hospital waiting rooms. It seems to be an unwritten rule of respect.

As I follow the tech, I am expecting to walk through the doors to the rooms across the hall. That's where the ultrasound rooms are located. I almost bump into her as she stopped and turned. "You can get dressed. We don't need any additional tests," she informed me. (Yeehaw, and thank the angels above!)

I am a bit giddy when I emerged in my street clothes through the 'special waiting room' threshold. I don't want to embarrass Tony with an alleluia dance, so I contain myself.

"Let's go," I announce. I watch his head lift up from the magazine and see the question in his eyes; he looked at me with big eyes.

"I'm good; all clear."

In the split second that it took him to register this 'turn of events,' I watched him take in a deep breath, let out a puff of air, and I saw then witnessed a release of stress move from his shoulders down to his feet. His body loosened and then his eyes welled up with tears.

"Really?" he asked.

"Yep," I replied, as I leaned over to kiss him.

He accepted it with a dazed look, making it a little peck on the lips. So I offered one more, and made this one last a bit longer. As we separated to look in each other's eyes, warmth between us, I added, "I suppose I should say, Happy Birthday?"

Yep, this gift was the best birthday present, ever.

# February 28
## Coffeee-Head

"Mom, have you been drinking a lot of coffee?" It's early in the morning. The boys have eaten breakfast, but the routine of smoothies has been changed to toast, so I didn't have my usual 'blender' alarm clock getting me out of bed. It was Tim and Gus, the dog, who burst through the door and rousted me up. I headed to the kitchen with a stiff hobble to pour a cup of hot water and was a bit confused by Matthias' morning greeting.

"Matthias. I drink tea. You know that. Why are you asking about coffee?" I glance at Tony, who is sitting at the table putting a spoonful of cereal into his mouth, and catch the amusement in his eyes. He isn't grinning, but rather is working at keeping a chuckle to himself.

"Your hair, Mom. It's sticking straight up. You know, like the people who drink too much coffee. That's what their hair looks like."

Lord knows where he got that image, but he's correct about mine. My 'bedhead' has the resemblance of a wavy 'fro.' It's resumed its original thickness, and though it's still short (I've cut it three times), I'm back to using a blow dryer before leaving on these below-zero February mornings. I still don't bother with hair spray; I suspect the bottle is gummed up from lack of use this past year.

I am getting stronger and am less fatigued at the end of my day with the 5/6 graders at Marine. A year ago, I was recovering from the removal of my appendix. Taking it one day at a time has made the weeks and months pass with gentle grace. For that, I am grateful!

My 'book' is in the hands of a copy-editor. For real. Really. It's really going to be published and available for any willing buyer. I am hopeful that it will benefit readers around the world - patients, survivors, family members, and their friends who experience the cancer challenges.

# June 21

## *Authors Assisted by Angels*

On my drive into Stillwater yesterday to run errands, I thought about last summer, just a year ago, when I made daily trips to New Richmond for radiation. Was it really me? Did I really have breast cancer? On the outside, I no longer have signs of cancer treatment. But I am changed.

And then I met Laura Sobiech for the first time, in Cub Foods, doing what is considered an everyday, normal task. And on the outside, no one would know what life has presented for her to endure. We don't carry battle scars, but then nor did the others who walked around us in the produce section. I suppose that is a good thing. But experiencing life's challenges with faith that there are angels by your side allows for a new understanding of subtle internal shifts in our essence. It may not be recognized in the normal settings of our lives, but the connectedness with one another on earth is apparent for some of us, in ways others may never experience. In the moment of a simple hug, surrounded by potatoes and tomatoes, I understood ours, Laura's and mine.

One day at a time, and life can shine through in writing and dancing, in songs and prayers. Angels watch over us all. :-) I'm so glad to have finally connected with the mom of Zach, who I've mentioned several times in this book.

There's a video on YouTube about Zach's family and friends called "One Year Later." You'll need 25 minutes and a box of kleenex to watch- but it's real stuff and worth the time.

Hugs to all.

https://www.youtube.com/watch?v=5iTImZGOtc4

# July 2014
## An Epilogue - Of Sorts

"And once the storm is over, you won't remember how you made it through, how you managed to survive. You won't even be sure, in fact, whether the storm is really over. But one thing is certain. When you come out of the storm, you won't be the same person who walked in." (Author Unknown)

As I purchased items at the Marine General Store one day this winter, one of the locals looked at me and exclaimed, "Is that hair yours? It is adorable!" At least she was looking at my head and face. Breast cancer patients learn to expect inquiries after a glance of the chest. "Are those real?" Hmmm, do you think the individual means God-given or man-made? Really, either way, they belong to us, altered or not. Just sayin'.

When the school year ended with students, I spent time with Dr. Amy. She added me into her busy schedule to remove my port on one of her Lakeview days. The procedure was done in an operating room under local anesthesia, which allowed the gals in scrubs and me to chatter. I always commented on how well she hid the little gadget in my breast tissue. She had to do some 'digging,' but once that bugger was out, I short of jumped off the table and danced down the hallway. No wheelchair for me - my energy level has returned to that of a 'normal' 55-year-old.

Much of my life has returned to normal. The neuropathy continued throughout the Herceptin infusions, but the pain in my feet is lessening. My hair has been cut many times, and Tim recently told me at the beach that I needed to 'shave down there.' Somehow I wasn't quite prepped enough for wearing swimsuit attire at the start of this summer. I am back to grabbing my tweezers in the van to pluck the stuff on my lip and chin as I drive. I did this on my way to my first author talk in Stillwater. Matthias recently told me I had a mustache and needed to shave, "Seriously, Mom." Geez, I can't say I am enjoying ripping the wax off my upper lip, again, but the irony of the hair growth has me chuckling.

As I reflect on last summer at the lake, I remember listening to the 4th of July fireworks from our bedroom window in our park model unit. All others at Mallard Lake Family Resort were on the beach watching the little display. I was too exhausted to consider walking down to join them. This year, I suggested to Tony that we spend time together in that same room, while the others 'oooed' and 'ahhhed' at the explosions in the sky. He made sure the boys were all set with friends for the event and joined me for a few fireworks of our own. With the exception of needing stuff and considering our age, we are doing just fine in that department. Celebrating the return of energy and better health can occur in many ways.

I never dreamed that my cancer road trip would lead to publishing a book, available as an e-reader download, in audio, and in good, old-fashioned paper versions. The boys shake their heads when we talk about the title of my book.

I told Tim while driving in the car. "Mom, that's awkward."

"Hey, buddy, you were the one who just asked me if I lost my vagina hair, your words, remember. People want to know."

When I told Matthias, he stood before me as I sat in a chair. It took a few seconds for the title to sink in, then he shook his head back and forth. "That's not a picture I want in my head!" he remarked.

"Well, don't think about it then," I suggested as he walked away.

In his philosophical manner, Tony said it was important for the boys to understand cancer treatment is more than just that question. It's about the many unknowns that this road trip leads you through.

Choose to celebrate your life. Each day, each moment, each breath, may you find purpose in them.

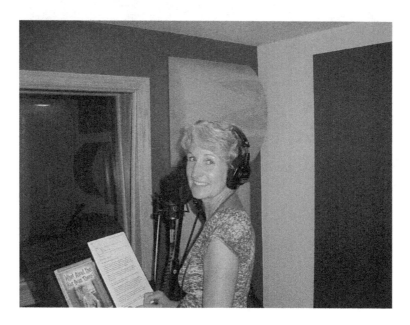

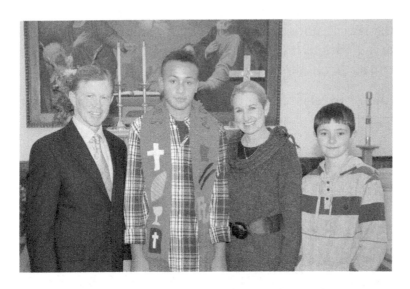

*Photo by Matt Mondor, Christ Lutheran Church, Marine on St. Croix, MN.*

# Acknowledgments

T his is the place to express deep gratitude for those who bring a book to publication. It wasn't an expectation that breast cancer would bring me here. I didn't keep a list of who to thank, but when I was diagnosed there was an outpouring of family and friends, from near and far, as well as community members who reached out in countless ways. Each one contributed to my emotional well-being during my cancer treatment. I can't name them all. Please know who you are and just how thankful I am that you are a part of my life.

Little did I imagine the ten-year-old, Kent Gustavson, 5th grader in my first class at Marine Elementary, would one day contact me to turn my Caring Bridge journal entries into a book for the masses. His successes don't surprise me though, and I am proud that he publishes Books That Matter through Blooming Twig. Contributing to our world in positive ways is part of his nature. Thanks, Young Sir!

The medical staff at Stillwater Medical Group, Lakeview Hospital, and New Richmond Radiology deserve kudos for professional, loving care. Most significantly, I need to thank Dr. Gary Williams for finding the lump (you saved my life), Dr. Amy Fox (the best bedside manner and surgeon around), and Dr. Candy Corey (even though you delivered the worst of the news!).

And the connectedness of my immediate family wove incredible support into this life's challenge. We have been through a few of them, Tony Brown; being your wife is an honor and privilege. You are one incredible husband.

The unconditional love of my parents, Art and Dianne Marquart, and siblings, Anne Bacigalupo and Kristine Kennelly, along with their families, helped me trudge forward with faith that all would be well. And a special gratefulness goes to the angels for you two, Matthias and Tim Brown. Without your unique personalities and perspectives as children of a mom with breast cancer, I wouldn't have nearly as much "funny stuff" to share with the readers. Thanks for being brave with me and taking it one day at a time.

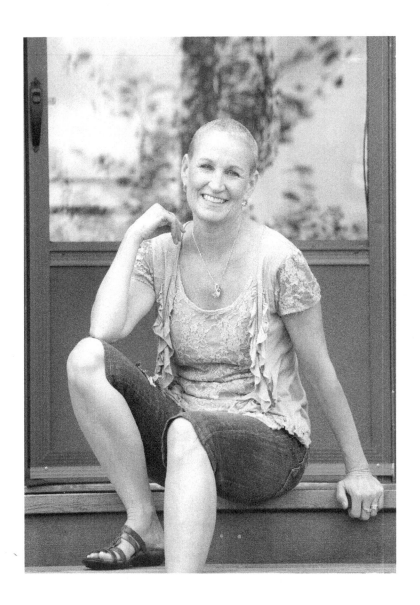

# About the Author

Abby Brown is an educator of twenty-five years, the mother of two teenaged boys, and a breast cancer survivor. She still spends her energy and days with fifth and sixth graders at her little grade school in Marine, Minnesota, a small town on the St. Croix River that most say is the place upon which Garrison Keillor based his fictional town of Lake Wobegon.

Abby made national news in 2009 with her "Stand Up for Learning" initiative, and her small school made front page headlines in the New York Times for its use of the now-patented Alphabetter Student Desk — an adjustable-height standing work station for students.

*"From the hallway, Abby Brown's sixth-grade classroom in a little school here about an hour northeast of Minneapolis has the look of the usual one, with an American flag up front and children's colorful artwork decorating the walls. But inside, an experiment is going on that makes it among the more unorthodox public school classrooms in the country, and pupils are being studied as much as they are studying. Unlike children almost everywhere, those in Ms. Brown's class do not have to sit and be still. Quite the contrary, they may stand and fidget all class long if they want."*

— From the NY Times article about Abby Brown and her classroom at Marine Elementary

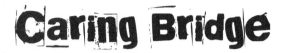

A portion of the proceeds of the sales of this book will go to support CaringBridge. Founded as a non-profit organization in 1997, CaringBridge enables healing during times of need through the support of family, friends and caregivers. Their mission states: "We work as the catalyst of love and healing for more than half a million people each day."

## What CaringBridge Offers

Personal, protected websites, free of advertising, including:

- Journals to share updates.
- Guestbooks to offer encouragement.
- A Planner tool to help coordinate life's daily logistics.

## How to Get Involved

*There are a number of ways to support the CaringBridge purpose.*

## Donating

CaringBridge is made possible through the compassion and generosity of people like you. There are a number of ways to make a tax-deductible contribution – from making a personal donation or giving in honor of a loved one to selecting CaringBridge as a beneficiary of your event or fundraiser.

## Volunteering

CaringBridge volunteers make such a significant impact in advancing the organization's mission that they don't just call them volunteers – they are called their "Amplifiers." Whether a CaringBridge Amplifier gives a few minutes or a few hours a month, it all goes a long way in enabling healing.

Visit **www.caringbridge.org** for more information.